# The 30-Minute

# AYURVEDIC
# COOKBOOK

## Healing Recipes for Total Wellness

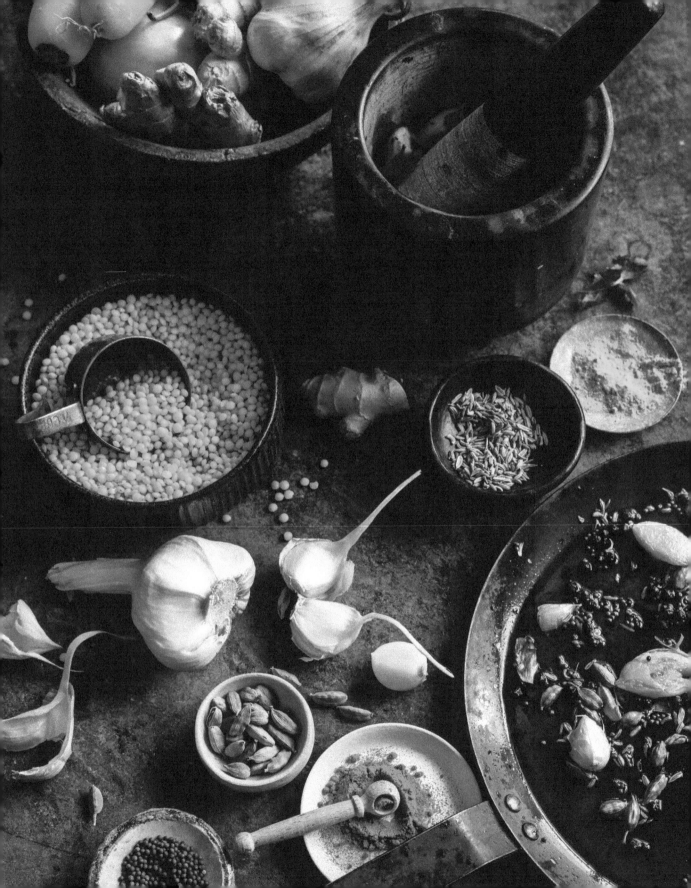

# The 30-Minute
# AYURVEDIC COOKBOOK

## Healing Recipes for Total Wellness

**Danielle Martin**

Photography by Annie Martin

ROCKRIDGE PRESS

For general information on our other products and services or to obtain technical support, please contact our Customer Care Department within the United States at (866) 744-2665, or outside the United States at (510) 253-0500.

Rockridge Press publishes its books in a variety of electronic and print formats. Some content that appears in print may not be available in electronic books, and vice versa.

Interior and Cover Designer: Amanda Kirk
Art Producer: Janice Ackerman
Editor: Samantha Barbaro
Production Editor: Mia Moran
Photography © 2019 Annie Martin. Food styling by Lukas Grossmann.
Author photo courtesy of James Martin

ISBN: Print 978-1-64611-123-7 | eBook 978-1-64611-124-4

R0

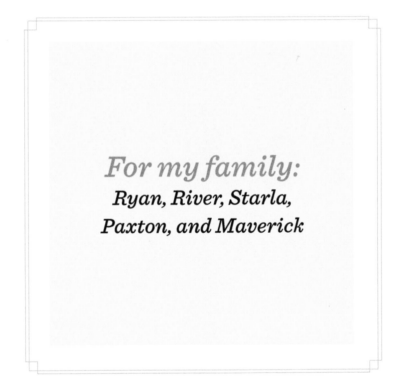

*For my family:*
**Ryan, River, Starla, Paxton, and Maverick**

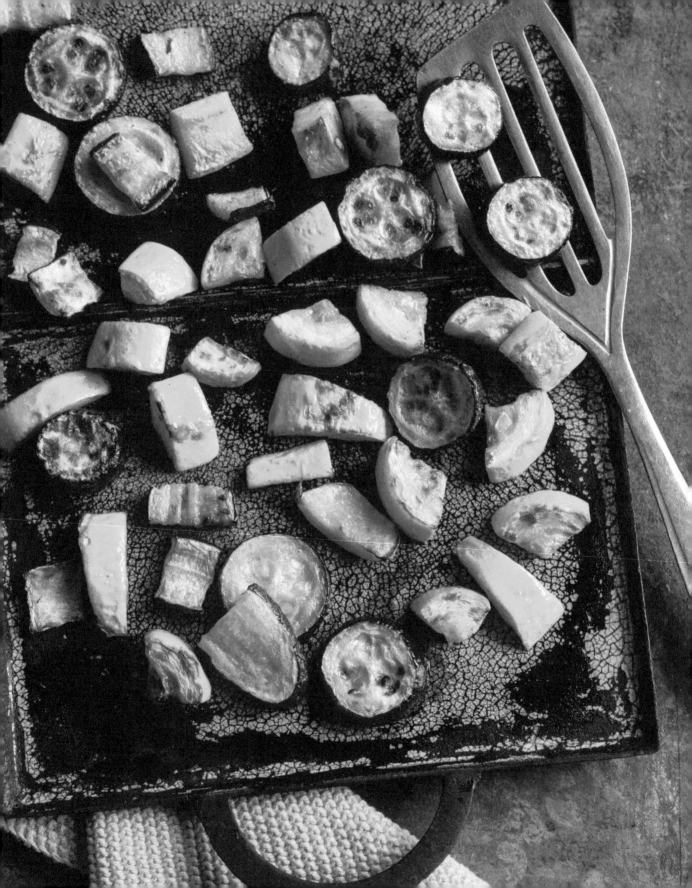

# CONTENTS

# INTRODUCTION
# + HOW TO USE
# THIS BOOK

**I** **first stumbled upon Ayurveda when studying Yoga back in 2007.**
I became so intrigued by it, I decided to continue my studies and
moved to New Mexico to enroll in the Ayurvedic Institute under
the renowned Dr. Vasant Lad. After graduating from his program, my
hunger for knowledge still burned strong. I discovered a traditional
school in Colorado and found myself moving once again to study
at Alandi Ayurveda Gurukula under the lovely Alakananda Ma and
passionate Dr. Bharat Vaidya. In 2013, I graduated from this four-year
program and embarked on a new path, putting my newly acquired
knowledge into action.

During my journey of studying both Yoga and Ayurveda, I not only
learned how to help others heal, but uncovered the healing process
I needed in my own life. This process included physical healing as well
as focusing on the mental, emotional, and spiritual. Although a per-
sonal journey is always a work in progress, Ayurveda blessed me with
the necessary tools to make a transformation, and to this day, I use
them to learn and to grow into my fullest potential.

One of the major lessons that Ayurveda has taught me is that we
are all unique beings with unique needs: What is healing for one, is not

healing for all. This resonated with me on a deep level, because I saw that determining what one needs really comes down to listening to your body. This profound revelation allowed me to home in on what was essential in my diet and lifestyle to reach a balanced state of health and maintain a high quality of life.

I am so grateful to be able to share this gift with others. The diet and health-care fads that are so prevalent online these days have only led to confusion and frustration, often doing more harm than good. With Ayurveda, a healthy diet is truly about going back to the basics and listening to your own innate intelligence and common sense.

As you read through this book, you will discover the basic principles of Ayurveda and how to use food choices to heal your body, mind, and consciousness. Your diet has the potential to bring you to a perfect state of health, and with these simple 30-minute recipes you can begin to find balance in your day-to-day life. Since many of us tend to live busy, on-the-go lifestyles, this book's focus is to make an Ayurvedic diet accessible to all by presenting healthy, delicious, and easy-to-make recipes. So take a deep breath and clear your mind as we walk down a new path of health, happiness—and good eating.

Sweet Potato Scramble Chapati Wrap **86**

# PART I

## Ayurveda and You

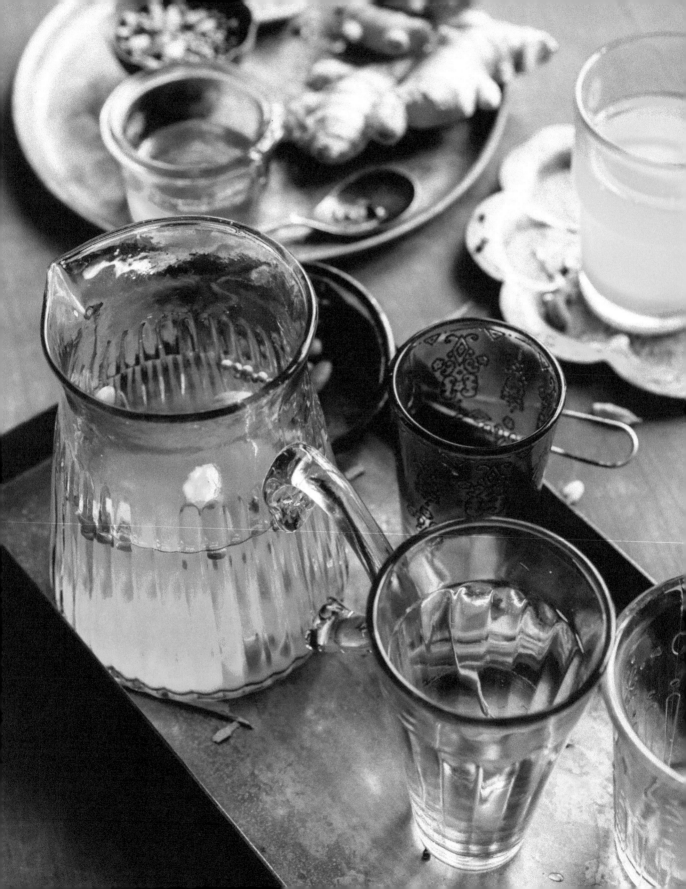

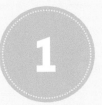

# ALL ABOUT AYURVEDA

An age-old medical science based on three doshas, five elements, and 20 main qualities, Ayurveda helps you cultivate awareness of your body and mind, and presents natural ways to bring balance back to your system. In this chapter, you'll get a brief overview of Ayurvedic history, how you can apply this ancient knowledge in the modern world, and how you can use Ayurveda to establish health and wellness in your life.

# What Is Ayurveda and What Does It Mean for Me?

Ayurveda is a medical, philosophical, and spiritual science that has been around for thousands of years. *Ayurveda* translates as the "science of life," but it more accurately means the science of finding balance, harmony, and peace in your life. Ayurveda empowers you to cultivate the self-awareness to know what you need as an individual to sustain a true sense of wellness. Ayurveda is strongly rooted in the idea that health is not just the absence of disease, but establishing complete harmony and happiness in body, mind, and soul.

Through the regular practice of Ayurveda, you can begin to create a sense of balance in your life. Proper diet and lifestyle practices allow you to increase your energy level, balance your emotions, prevent future illness, and heal current disorders. Once you find your dosha, you can home in on the common foods and habits that will either bring you health or cause "dis-ease." By becoming familiar with the principles of Ayurveda, you will build a strong foundation on your journey to a self-empowered, holistic way of living.

## An Ancient Science

Ayurveda originated 5,000 years ago from the great *rishis* (sages) of India while they were deep in meditation. Considered the first established medical system, its wisdom still holds true today. This science was passed down through an oral tradition and eventually written in the great classical texts. Although these great *vaidyas* (doctors) before us did not have medical technology or clinical trials, they came to many of the very same findings Western medicine is only just discovering today.

## Ayurveda Today

Ayurveda is considered a living science. This means that although Ayurveda was discovered thousands of years ago, with some modifications you can still apply its basic principles to your modern-day needs. For example, you will notice that many recipes in this book are neither traditionally Ayurvedic nor from Indian culture; however, they are still considered Ayurvedic as long as you follow the main dietary guidelines. With such essential principles as using whole food ingredients, incorporating Ayurvedic spices, eating for the season, and eating for your dosha type, you can modify *any* food or recipe to become Ayurvedic.

## 30-Minute Ayurveda

Creating an Ayurvedic diet and lifestyle can seem complicated, time-consuming, and overwhelming. In this book you will find simple recipes that can be created in 30 minutes or less, prep time included. To achieve this time limit, you may have to use precooked food and canned food, or make large batches of food to carry you through your busy week. While such preparation is not 100 percent aligned with traditionally Ayurvedic principles, the main intent still holds true: By making these recipes you can begin to adopt a healthy Ayurvedic diet in a realistic way. As you will learn, Ayurveda is not black or white, all or nothing!

## Ayurveda and Healing

Healing lies at the root of an Ayurvedic diet. Ayurveda can help you uncover the areas of your health that need attention, whether it's a small imbalance or a full-blown disease. This ancient science gives you the knowledge, clarity, and awareness to identify your imbalances, and then helps you break down those imbalances into tangible concepts and determine the best path for healing.

By following the wisdom of your dosha, you can adopt the diet and lifestyle practices that will bring you into balance. All the recipes in this book have been created to reduce the impact of an imbalanced dosha, as well as aid in easing specific issues such as digestive distress, anemia, inflammation, sleep disturbances, weight issues, toxin overload, and anxiety. Each recipe is labeled to help guide you in the right direction and can become a part of your meal rotation without becoming too time-consuming.

## Remedies and Recipes for Your Dosha

A dosha is a subtle, energetic, biological force that governs your actions, physical characteristics, personality, emotions, and mental functioning. There are three doshas, known as Kapha, Pitta, and Vata, that reside in the body. Each dosha is composed of two of the five main elements (earth, water, fire, air, and ether). Each dosha possesses unique qualities that reflect its respective elements. For example:

 **Kapha,** full of earth and water, tends to be slow, sluggish, sedentary, emotional, compassionate, loving, and nurturing.

 **Pitta,** made up of fire and water, tends to be hot, fiery, sharp, oily, determined, ambitious, angry, and critical.

 **Vata,** comprised of air and space, tends to be mobile, restless, imaginative, spacey, forgetful, light, cold, and dry.

The doshas also correlate to the seasons. By keeping the time of year in mind, you will know which dosha is most likely to be out of balance:

♦ **The winter and spring seasons** are known as the seasons of Kapha, causing conditions such as colds, cough, allergies, congestion, and weight gain to arise. By following a Kapha-balancing diet during these months you can avoid these common issues.

♦ **The late spring, summer, and early fall** are considered the seasons of Pitta due to their hot, sharp, and penetrating nature. This means that a Pitta diet should be followed, because Pitta episodes such as rash, acne, eczema, inflammation, anger, and loose stools tend to become more prevalent at this time.

♦ **The fall and early winter seasons** are related to Vata due to their dark, dry, windy, and cold qualities. Therefore, a Vata diet should be followed to avoid common Vata issues such as anxiety, insomnia, dry skin, gas, and constipation.

Understanding your dosha is essential for determining which foods, recipes, and remedies to favor and which to avoid. Let's move on to a quick quiz to reveal your main dosha. Before you begin, keep in mind that everyone possesses all three doshas, although their strength and ratio will vary. If you have a tendency toward more than one of the answers in this quiz, select the answer that pertains most strongly and has been most consistent throughout your life.

# WHAT'S MY DOSHA?

**What best describes your body frame?**

1. Small bone structure, fragile
2. Medium body frame, strong
3. Large bone structure, solid

**What best describes your body weight?**

1. Underweight
2. Average weight
3. Overweight

**What best describes your skin type?**

1. Dry, flaky, cold
2. Oily, pinkish, fair, warm
3. Oily, pale, cool, and clammy

**What best describes your eyes?**

1. Small, beady
2. Medium, almond shaped
3. Large and round

**What best describes your hair?**

1. Rough, dry, frizzy
2. Fine, oily, thinning, graying prematurely
3. Thick, oily, strong

**What best describes your appetite?**

1. Irregular, forget to eat, hunger fluctuates, spacey with hunger
2. Strong, cannot miss a meal, cranky with hunger
3. Dull, skip meals often, rarely hungry

**What best describes your digestion habits?**

1. Weak digestion, gas, bloating, cramping
2. Strong digestion, fast metabolism, acid reflux, inflammation
3. Slow digestion, poor metabolism, sleepy after food

**What best describes your sleep habits?**

1. Light sleeper, restless, difficulty falling asleep, anxious dreams
2. Medium sleeper, difficulty staying asleep; angry, fiery, or work-related dreams
3. Heavy sleeper, easy to fall and stay asleep, hard to wake; soft, pleasant, watery dreams

*continued on next page*

## What best describes your emotions?

1. Anxiety, worry, fear, fluctuating
2. Anger, irritation, judgmental, passionate
3. Sadness, depression, cry easily, repress emotions

## What best describes your mind?

1. Restless, distracted, creative, imaginative, forgetful, spacey
2. Sharp, quick-witted, perfectionist, critical thinker, sharp memory, debater
3. Dull, foggy, slow in thought and speech, agreeable, more follower than leader

## What best describes your temperament?

1. Active, talkative, imaginative, crave change, flighty, silly, indecisive
2. Serious, honest, loyal, hardworking, passionate, strong-willed, "all-or-nothing" attitude, decisive
3. Laid-back, slow but steady, patient, nurturing, compassionate, loving, soft-natured

## ANSWER KEY

**If you answered mostly:**

1, your dosha is Vata

2, your dosha is Pitta

3, your dosha is Kapha

**If you answered mostly:**

1 and secondly 2, your dosha is Vata with Pitta secondary

1 and secondly 3, your dosha is Vata with Kapha secondary

2 and secondly 1, your dosha is Pitta with Vata secondary

2 and secondly 3, your dosha is Pitta with Kapha secondary

3 and secondly 1, your dosha is Kapha with Vata secondary

3 and secondly 2, your dosha is Kapha with Pitta secondary

**If you answered equally:**

1 and 2, you are dual-doshic Vata-Pitta

1 and 3, you are dual-doshic Vata-Kapha

2 and 3, you are dual-doshic Pitta-Kapha

1, 2, and 3, you are tridoshic

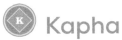 # Kapha

Kapha is the dosha made of water and earth elements, making these individuals strong, solid, and stable. Kapha types dislike arguments and, due to their watery nature, are very good at going with the flow. They are very heart-driven and as a result of this openness can be quite emotional, crying often and easily. They are overall slow in movement, speech, and thought. Physical characteristics include large, round eyes, thick, strong hair, porcelainlike skin, and melodious voices.

## Kapha in Alignment

When in balance, Kapha types display many great characteristics. They are compassionate, caring, nurturing beings loved by everyone they meet. They are easygoing and get along with others. They are loyal friends and great listeners. They are slow in movement and prefer to be sedentary, although once they get the motivation to move, they are able to keep an ongoing, steady pace. Balanced Kaphas often crave spicy, bitter, and astringent foods, all of which promote a healthy metabolism for their type.

## Kapha out of Alignment

Due to a prolonged Kapha-provoking diet, heavy in dairy, carbs, sweets, and meat, or an ongoing Kapha-increasing lifestyle consisting of sedentary daily living, daytime sleeping, lack of exercise, constant grazing, and eating late into the night, a person's constitution can lean too heavily in the sedentary direction. When Kapha is high, one may experience poor motivation, low energy, lethargy, and general sluggishness. There may be feelings of heaviness, a dull appetite, a slow metabolism, sleepiness after food, and weight gain. An individual may steer toward emotional eating and crave sweet and salty foods, both of which further provoke Kapha qualities. High Kapha can also result in such psychological effects as a dull, foggy mind, grief, sadness, depression, and attachment.

## Common Kapha Ailments

Increased Kapha for a prolonged amount of time can result in disorders. Some common Kapha ailments likely to occur include cold, cough, congestion, chronic sinus infections, allergies, weight issues, obesity, high cholesterol, high blood pressure, diabetes, and hypothyroidism. If Kapha is high in the mind, a person may become depressed, experience severe grief, and acquire a general sense of hopelessness. If you are experiencing any of these issues, you can benefit from incorporating Kapha-reducing recipes into your meal plan.

## Pitta

Pitta types are naturally hot, fiery, and passionate individuals. They are often fair-skinned, with light blond or red hair, sharp, piercing eyes, and medium body weight. Due to the excessive heat that accumulates in the head, they often tend toward baldness and premature graying. Pitta individuals love to learn, study, and solve problems, making them great professors, engineers, architects, and accountants. They are extremely goal-driven, disciplined, focused, organized, and dedicated, and often end up in high positions such as president, CEO, or any position of power, money, name, and fame. Due to their intense nature, Pitta types can become overly critical, judgmental, hot-tempered, self-absorbed, overworked, and high-strung if they are not careful. Many perfectionists and type A individuals fall in the Pitta category.

### Pitta in Alignment

A Pitta in balance possesses many great qualities. Being predominant in the fire element allows Pittas to be focused, driven, disciplined, and ambitious, leading them to great success in everything they do. Pitta types are witty and smart by nature and are always hungry for more knowledge. When in balance, Pitta types are loyal, courageous, charismatic, and natural leaders. They are great at motivating others, because people often look up to them and love to be around them. A Pitta in balance tends to crave sweet, bitter, and astringent foods, which align with what that body type needs to feel nourished.

### Pitta out of Alignment

Due to a prolonged Pitta-provoking diet, consisting of spicy, fatty, fried, fermented, and/or inflammatory foods, or an ongoing Pitta-increasing lifestyle made up of excessive sun exposure, overworking, ambition, excessively critical thinking, and high stress, Pitta can go out of balance in one's constitution. When this occurs, an individual may experience such issues as a short temper, extreme frustration and irritation, jealousy, and an overly judgmental attitude. Some physical issues that may arise include inflammation, redness, rash, acne, eczema, psoriasis, headaches, migraines, and liver conditions. Excessive Pitta in digestion may result in cranky hunger, hyper-metabolism, low blood sugar, and hyperacidity. Pitta types that are out of balance often crave spicy, salty, and sour foods, all of which exacerbate issues.

## Common Pitta Ailments

With increased Pitta, multiple disorders can emerge. Common Pitta digestive conditions include loose stools, hyperacidity, gastroesophageal reflux disease (GERD), heartburn, gastritis, colitis, diverticulitis, irritable bowel syndrome (IBS), and Crohn's disease. Since Pitta is intimately related to the skin, almost all skin conditions have an elevated Pitta origin, including acne, rash, hives, eczema, psoriasis, and rosacea. Pitta also correlates to the liver and eyes, and therefore all disorders related to these organs will have some involvement of high Pitta. When Pitta becomes out of balance in the mind, a person is likely to experience piercing headaches, migraines, hair loss, premature graying, sleep disturbances, anger, and irritation. If you are experiencing any of these conditions, it will be beneficial for you to follow a Pitta-reducing diet.

# Vata

Born from the elements air and ether, Vata individuals are creative, imaginative, talkative, energetic, and enthusiastic. Although they excel at coming up with new ideas and dreams, Vata types rarely accomplish them. They love to move and crave change. They bore easily with routine and find it hard to remain focused on any one particular task. As much as they dislike routine, having a set daily schedule is one of the best things for keeping Vata in balance. Vata types tend to have low body weight and can find it difficult to gain weight. Most have dry skin, dry hair, overactive minds, and overactive metabolisms. Vata is cold by nature; therefore, Vata individuals tend to chill easily, have poor circulation, and complain of cold hands and feet. Due to their restless nature, Vata types often experience racing thoughts, distracted concentration, difficulty sleeping, excessive worry, anxiety, fear, and indecisiveness.

## Vata in Alignment

When Vata is healthy and in balance, great qualities arise, such as creativity, optimal energy, and enthusiasm. When Vata is in alignment, these animated individuals have the ability to become great artists, dancers, writers, and actors.

Since Vata types love change, they go with the flow and adapt to what is needed. Vata types tend to be talkative and make friends easily. They are often seen as fun, silly, and playful, making them exciting and pleasant to be around. Healthy Vata individuals have amazing dreams, ideas, and imaginations, and when in balance they can envision—and create—great things.

## Vata out of Alignment

Due to a prolonged Vata-provoking diet filled with raw, cold, dry, and rough foods, as well as a Vata-increasing lifestyle that lacks routine or stability, one can experience symptoms of high Vata such as poor concentration, a hyperactive mind, excessive worry and fear, anxiety, and insecurity. Vata lives in the colon, which means high Vata often results in a person having gas, bloating, and constipation issues, along with weak, irregular appetite and digestion. When Vata becomes hyperactive, an individual may find it difficult to stick to a task and may change goals, jobs, homes, partners, and friends frequently. For someone with a restless mind and a restless body, high Vata is quick to create sleep disorders and often results in a person experiencing difficulty falling asleep, staying asleep, and quieting the mind at night.

## Common Vata Ailments

If Vata is increased for a long time, Vata disorders are sure to arise. Insomnia, attention-deficit/hyperactivity disorder (ADHD), severe anxiety, phobias, and most neurological disorders come from high Vata. One of the most common Vata conditions is constipation and often goes hand in hand with gas, bloating, belching, cramping, and intestinal gurgling. Since Vata is intimately related to the bones, osteoporosis, arthritis, and cracking, popping joints are all born from increased Vata. With dryness being one of the main qualities of Vata, dry, brittle skin, hair, and nails can result with excess in this dosha. Being light and fragile by nature, long-term high Vata is likely to cause low body weight, depletion, poor immunity, scanty menstruation, amenorrhea, infertility, and reduced libido. If you are experiencing a number of these Vata conditions, following a Vata-reducing diet is ideal.

# Blended Doshas and Being Tridoshic

It is fairly common for a person to be predominant in more than one dosha; however, it can lead to confusion regarding the best diet and lifestyle recommendations one should follow. Each dosha possesses unique qualities, many of which seem to oppose each other, making these concepts even more difficult to understand. Although being predominant in multiple doshas may take a bit more thought, that situation can actually be beneficial, because these doshas all have great aspects that can work together to strengthen your overall constitution.

There are three dual-doshic (equal in two doshas) combinations possible: Vata-Pitta, Vata-Kapha, and Pitta-Kapha. It is also possible to be tridoshic, meaning you are equal in all three doshas, but this is a rare occurrence. Although each manifestation of a blended dosha is unique, there is some common ground to consider when looking to balance multiple forces.

You will want to take into account the current season, climate, and overall environment of your area. Generally speaking, you will want to reduce Kapha for winter and spring, Pitta for summer, and Vata for fall.

You will also want to determine your current imbalances and which dosha is the cause of them. For example, if you are Vata-Pitta but suffer from anxiety, insomnia, and constipation, following a Vata-soothing diet proves the best. If you are Vata-Kapha but suffer from weight gain, slow metabolism, depression, and lethargy, adopting a Kapha-reducing diet will be essential. By breaking down all the determining factors, you can simplify these complicated areas. And if all else fails, follow the tridoshic recommendations for a safe alternative!

## Vata-Pitta

Vata and Pitta are both light and mobile by nature; therefore, foods, drinks, and spices that are considered heavy and grounding benefit both doshas. Pitta and Vata are similarly pacified by the sweet taste and therefore sweet, soothing foods such as dates, ripe mango, sweet juicy fruits, maple syrup, rice, wheat, and dairy are great options for both. Additional beneficial food and spice options include fresh ginger, turmeric, fennel, cardamom, ghee, mung dal, red lentils, quinoa, oats, buckwheat, sweet potato, carrots, zucchini, squash, hemp seeds, pumpkin seeds, and almonds. Because both Vata and Pitta are provoked by nightshades, it's best to limit tomatoes, potatoes, peppers, and eggplant.

If you are a Vata-Pitta type, it may be helpful for you to eat with the seasons by following a Pitta diet and lifestyle during the summer and then switching to a Vata-reducing diet and lifestyle throughout the fall. During the winter and spring seasons, you can follow a Kapha-reducing diet; however, if your Vata or Pitta is out of balance, it's best to favor the dosha diet that best aligns the imbalance.

## Vata-Kapha

Vata and Kapha may seem like opposites, but the common denominator is their cold quality. This means that warming foods, drinks, spices, and herbs will be best for the Vata-Kapha body type to pacify these forces. Vata and Kapha tend to have weak digestion, and although their symptoms manifest differently, they both benefit from easy-to-digest meals, and warming, digestion-enhancing spices and herbs.

If you are a Vata-Kapha type, it may be helpful for you to eat with the seasons by following a Vata diet and lifestyle during the fall, and switching to a Kapha-reducing diet and lifestyle throughout the winter and spring. During the summer season, you can follow a Pitta-reducing diet; however, if your Kapha or Vata is out of balance, it's best to favor the dosha diet that best aligns the imbalance.

## Pitta-Kapha

Pitta and Kapha share the common trait of being oily by nature, and therefore both types favor drying foods, drinks, and spices. Since Pitta is hot and Kapha is cold, it will be best to choose neutral or warm foods and spices to find a middle ground. Beneficial foods include quinoa, buckwheat, mung dal, red lentils, chickpeas, ghee, sunflower oil, zucchini, yellow squash, kale, bitter greens, celery, lime, and almonds. Beneficial spices include fresh ginger, fennel, cumin, turmeric, and cardamom.

If you are a Pitta-Kapha type, it may be helpful for you to eat with the seasons by following a Pitta diet and lifestyle during the summer, and then switching to a Kapha-reducing diet and lifestyle throughout the winter and spring. During the fall season, you can follow a Vata-reducing diet; however, if your Pitta or Kapha is out of balance, it's best to favor the dosha diet that best aligns the imbalance.

## Tridoshic

Being tridoshic (equal in all three doshas) is an unlikely occurrence. According to Dr. Vasant Lad of the Ayurvedic Institute, it is so rare for an individual to be born tridoshic, that in his 50-plus years as an Ayurvedic doctor, he has personally never come across it. A blessed tridoshic individual experiences completely balanced digestion, elimination, emotions, mental functioning, energy, and overall health. They are indeed enlightened by nature.

If your results show that you are equal in all three doshas, this more likely states that you have a strong presence with all three doshas, although one may be slightly less than the other two. However, all things considered, you will still want to follow a tridoshic diet and lifestyle program, making sure to welcome foods, drinks, and daily habits that are beneficial for all three doshas. Some great food and spice options include fresh ginger, turmeric, fennel, coriander, cardamom, ghee, almonds, pumpkin seeds, hemp seeds, quinoa, buckwheat, egg whites, mung beans, red lentils, zucchini, yellow squash, carrots, cilantro, and lime.

In general, eating with the seasons will be beneficial for you by following a Kapha-reducing diet and lifestyle during the winter and spring seasons, a Pitta diet and lifestyle during the summer, and a Vata-reducing diet and lifestyle throughout the fall. However, if any one dosha seems out of balance, it's best to favor the dosha diet that best aligns the imbalance.

Now that you have learned a bit about Ayurveda, let's move on to discover how to heal through an Ayurveda-based diet. In the following chapters, you'll find Ayurvedic principles of eating, how to eat for your dosha, and how to incorporate these guidelines into your life in a stress-free manner.

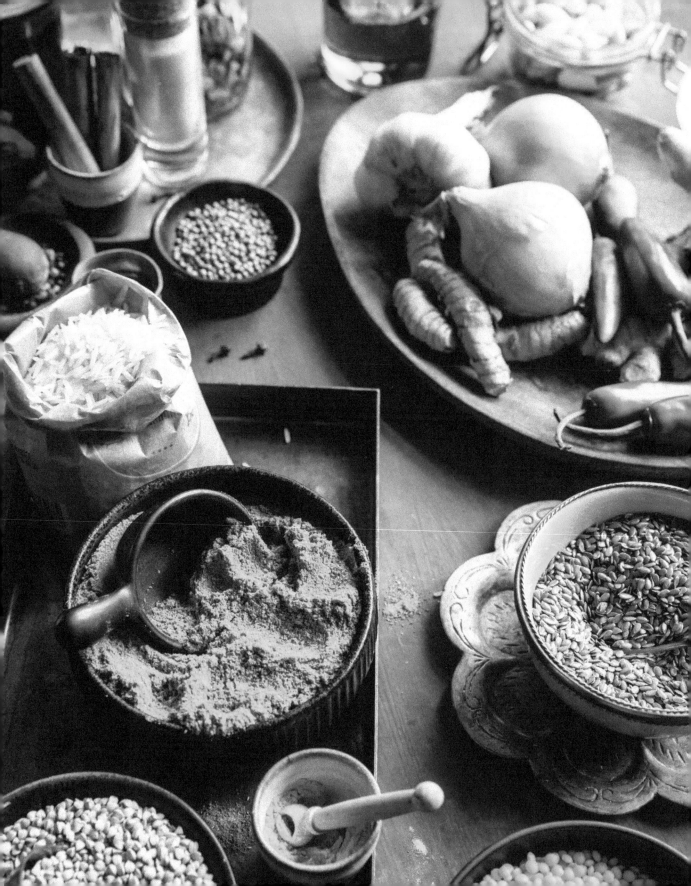

# 30-MINUTE AYURVEDIC EATING

An Ayurvedic diet plan means eating for your specific body type, as well as for the appropriate season. Now that you have discovered your dosha, you can understand how to stay in balance and heal from disease through your food choices. In this chapter, I have laid out realistic, sustainable ways to keep up an Ayurvedic meal plan. Keep in mind that Ayurveda is not just black or white, but should be thought of as a spectrum. Plenty of modifications can be made to allow for flexibility without compromising the healing nature of Ayurveda. Keep reading to discover the main principles of an Ayurvedic diet and a realistic approach to incorporating these principles into your life.

# When and What You Eat

According to Ayurveda, the root cause of all disease starts with improper digestion, and healthy digestion signals optimal health. By setting up a consistent meal schedule that follows the proper times, proper foods, and the proper quantities to eat, you can begin to strengthen your digestion.

Once you establish a routine meal schedule, you'll begin to notice positive changes. Having a balanced breakfast provides you with energy throughout the morning and keeps hunger at bay until lunchtime. Having a large—but healthy—lunch midday allows you to refuel, keeping your energy and mental focus high and bright. Ending your day with an early, light dinner supplies you with the nourishment you need before bed without triggering indigestion or sleep disturbances.

Did you know that your digestion relies on routine to maintain its strength and vitality? Just as a fire goes out when it no longer has wood to burn, skipping meals or eating too late weakens your digestive fire. When you establish a consistent and healthy meal schedule, your digestion continuously burns strong as it is replenished when needed without being suffocated (by overeating) or starved (by eating too little). Once you set the routine, your digestive fire becomes familiar with these mealtimes, and naturally becomes stimulated before each meal as it prepares to receive food. With so many digestive disorders affecting so many people, making this one small change can make a big impact!

## Mealtimes

Here are some general recommendations for mealtimes and the qualities to aim for in each meal.

| Time | Meal | Qualities |
|------|------|-----------|
| 6:00 a.m. to 8:00 a.m. | Breakfast | Medium in size; filled with whole grains, fiber, and lean protein |
| 11:00 a.m. to 1:00 p.m. | Lunch | Largest, most nourishing meal of the day; favor lean protein, colorful veggies, and high-fiber foods; best time to eat heavier foods such as meat and dairy |
| 5:00 p.m. to 7:00 p.m. | Dinner | Light, easy-to-digest meal; favor simple foods such as soups, kitchari, and stir-fries; avoid heavy foods such as meat, dairy, pasta, bread, refined grains, simple sugars, and heavy carbs |

Sometimes your schedule simply won't accommodate this routine. If so, it's okay to make some adjustments. For example, let's say you regularly return from work around 9:00 p.m. The best option is to bring a light, healthy meal into work, and take a dinner break before 7:00 p.m. each night. For some, this is still not possible. In that case, I recommend eating a light, extra-simple, already-prepared meal when you get home. Instead of following each guideline to the letter, it's best (and most realistic) for you to keep the guidelines in mind as you adjust them to your schedule.

### Snacking

Snacking is not typically recommended in an Ayurvedic diet. However, it's sometimes necessary to refuel between meals to make it through a busy day. Fortunately, like most matters in Ayurveda, the "no snacking" rule can be modified to meet your needs! When considering a healthy snack, keep this in mind:

- Avoid grazing; snacks should be kept small, simple, and healthy.

- Avoid snacking on the go; eat snacks while sitting down and with full awareness.

- Wait two to three hours after a meal before snacking.

- Avoid snacking after dinner and/or late-night snacking.

## Eating for Balance

It is no secret that proper foods can help you gain energy, strength, clarity, and overall wellness, whereas improper food choices can lead to indigestion, lethargy, toxicity, and ailments. There are many factors to consider when deciding which foods will be best for you.

If you are feeling overwhelmed about food choices, begin with your dosha. Each dosha has specific foods to help bring you into balance—as well as foods that will likely aggravate your system. Knowing your predominant dosha allows you to focus on foods and recipes that are beneficial for your body type, and helps you limit those that can cause imbalance. As you will see, foods that are healing for some people can have adverse effects for others.

**Kapha**—Because of the heavy, dense, oily, and slow qualities associated with Kapha, it is imperative these individuals avoid food with similar qualities. Some foods to limit include heavy meats (such as red meat and pork), dairy, carb-rich foods, refined grains, and excessive sweets because they can increase Kapha and result in lethargy, mental fogginess, weight gain, and a slow metabolism. If you are Kapha, aim to consume foods that are considered light, drying, and stimulating, such as hot-spicy foods, vegetables, light whole grains (quinoa and millet), and lots of stimulating digestive spices. Eating a diet rich in these foods reduces the characteristics of Kapha, bringing balance to your system.

**Pitta**—Naturally hot, sharp, and fiery, Pitta types will want to reduce their intake of foods that hold similar qualities because these foods can contribute to eczema, acne, rash, hyperacidity, anger, irritability, and frustration. If you are Pitta, you will want to avoid hot-spicy, fermented, fatty-fried, sour, and inflammatory foods (such as red meat, nightshades, and refined sugar). When aiming to find balance, you should favor cooling, soothing foods such as sweet fruits, coconut, ghee, milk, basmati rice, cilantro, juicy vegetables, bitter greens, and aloe. By knowing these simple rules, you can begin to reduce the heat in your system.

**Vata**—Vata is light, dry, and cold by nature; therefore, foods that carry these properties increase Vata (like increases like). Vata types should avoid cold, dry, and raw foods such as green juices, cold smoothies, crackers, dry cereals, and raw vegetables because they increase symptoms such as gas, bloating, constipation, dryness, spaciness, anxiety, and insomnia. If you are Vata, you should choose grounding foods that are heavy, moist, oily, and warming. Some classic examples of Vata-balancing foods include basmati rice, soups, stews, casseroles, porridges, and oatmeal. Following a diet with these guidelines will be essential for calming your Vata.

# The Six Tastes of Ayurveda

According to Ayurveda, there are six essential tastes to include in your diet: sweet, sour, salty, pungent (spicy), bitter, and astringent. Your health relies on getting a balance of each taste in your daily diet, because each flavor possesses different healing properties. Here is an overview:

| Taste | Energy | Health Properties |
|---|---|---|
| SWEET | Cooling | Energizes; promotes rejuvenation, strength, longevity, happiness, contentment, nourishment, love, and compassion |
| SOUR | Heating | Stimulates the appetite, digestion, and metabolism; energizes; awakens the mind; reduces gas and bloating |
| SALTY | Heating | Improves flavor of food; enhances digestion, absorption, and elimination; reduces gas and bloating; maintains electrolyte balance; increases energy, strength, and enthusiasm |
| PUNGENT (SPICY) | Heating | Increases digestion and metabolism; burns toxins; increases circulation; removes congestion; increases energy; promotes clarity, focus, and concentration |
| BITTER | Cooling | Improves all other tastes; detoxifies; reduces heat in the liver and blood; is antibacterial; is anti-inflammatory; reduces blood sugar levels; is beneficial for the skin; reduces sweet cravings |
| ASTRINGENT | Cooling | Improves absorption of nutrients; is beneficial in diarrhea; reduces heat and inflammation; removes congestion; increases dryness; reduces fat and cholesterol; detoxifies |

**Dosha Taste Chart**

| Taste | Best for | Food Sources |
|---|---|---|
| SWEET | Pitta, Vata | Honey, maple syrup, banana, coconut, sweet potato, milk, rice, wheat |
| SOUR | Vata | Citrus, pineapple, strawberries, vinegar, fermented foods |
| SALTY | Vata | Mineral salt, sea salt, table salt, seaweed, soy sauce |
| PUNGENT | Kapha | Cayenne pepper, chiles, black pepper, garlic, onion, ginger |
| BITTER | Kapha, Pitta | Kale, collard greens, coffee, tea, cacao |
| ASTRINGENT | Kapha, Pitta | Pomegranate, aloe, unripe bananas, beans, lentils, raw vegetables |

## The 20 Qualities of Ayurveda

A basic principle of Ayurveda states that everything—including your food—possesses unique qualities that have a specific effect on your body. There are 20 main qualities to know about when you are striving for health and balance. By becoming familiar with these qualities, you can see the impact they have on your health and you can begin to decide which foods are beneficial for you and which to limit or avoid.

Again, if your system is skewed in one direction, you can find balance by avoiding foods with similar properties and favoring foods with the opposite qualities. For example, if you are experiencing too much heaviness, opt for light foods and limit heavy foods. If you have too much heat, welcome in more cooling foods and hold off on warming foods.

| Quality | Good for | Foods |
|---|---|---|
| COLD | Pitta | Aloe, cucumber, lime, cilantro, kale, lettuce, watermelon, zucchini, asparagus, pomegranate |
| HOT | Kapha, Vata | Ginger, chiles, black pepper, salt, lemon juice |
| LIGHT | Kapha | Sprouts, lettuce, raw vegetables, apples, toast, broth, soup |
| HEAVY | Pitta, Vata | Dairy, meat, wheat, rice, pasta, bread, whole grains |
| OILY | Vata | Ghee, nuts, seeds, coconut, avocado, olive oil, sesame oil |
| DRY | Kapha | Crackers, dry toast, pretzels, rice cakes, raw vegetables |
| SLIMY | Pitta, Vata | Cheese, dairy, white rice, oats, licorice, okra |
| ROUGH | Kapha | Raw vegetables, crackers, dry toast, rice cakes, dry cereal, granola, pretzels |
| SLOW/DULL | Pitta, Vata | High-carb foods, white rice, meat, dairy, wheat, oats, pasta |
| SHARP | Kapha | Cayenne pepper, black pepper, ginger, chiles, lemon juice |

| Quality | Good for | Foods |
| --- | --- | --- |
| SOFT | Pitta, Vata | White rice, bread, pasta, soft cheese, yogurt, dairy |
| HARD | Kapha | Raw vegetables, crackers, dry toast, rice cakes, dry cereal, granola |
| DENSE | Pitta, Vata | Dairy, meat, wheat, tofu, sweet potato, starchy foods |
| LIQUID | Vata | Water, healthy oils, juicy fruits, watery vegetables |
| STATIC | Pitta, Vata | Dairy, meat, wheat, tofu, sweet potato, pasta, bread |
| MOBILE | Kapha | Raw juice, raw vegetables, sprouts, caffeine, alcohol, cacao |
| GROSS | Pitta, Vata | Dairy, meat, wheat, rice, high-carb foods, starchy foods, sweet potato, tofu, bread, pasta |
| SUBTLE | Kapha | Raw juice, raw vegetables, sprouts, alcohol, caffeine, chiles, ginger, salt |
| CLEAR | Kapha | Raw juice, raw vegetables, sprouts, alcohol, caffeine |
| CLOUDY | Pitta, Vata | Yogurt, milk, cheese, sugar, sweets, yeast, ice cream |

## Non-Ayurvedic Foods to Avoid

Although I often say any food can be Ayurvedic, I am referring to unprocessed whole foods. Unfortunately, multiple "fake" foods have made their way into our regular diets. Here are the foods you should avoid altogether, and a few others you should greatly limit.

### Completely Avoid:

- Deli meat
- Fast food
- GMOs (e.g., many soy and corn products; products with white sugar)
- Honey that has been heated to over 110°F
- Hydrogenated oils (e.g., vegetable oil, shortening, margarine)
- "Low-fat," "reduced fat," or "fat-free" foods (e.g., low-fat yogurt or fat-free milk)
- Soda and sugary drinks
- Sugar substitutes that contain aspartame
- White sugar (found in most candy, ice cream, baked goods, and sugary beverages)

### Limit:

- Canned foods
- Eating out
- Frozen foods
- Ice cream
- Processed foods
- Refined grains

If this list seems overwhelming, don't worry! Take these changes in stride, and make one or two changes at a time. If you have multiple foods you need to eliminate, begin by choosing one that is fairly common in your diet and slowly wean yourself off it. For example, if you are eating ice cream every night, begin by cutting back to every other night. After a week or so, reduce this even further by making it a weekend-only treat. After you've accomplished this, you can move on to having a bowl as a special occasion once a month or so. Just remember: Major changes don't happen overnight, so it is important to practice patience and self-compassion as you move forward.

## When and What to Drink

When it comes to a healthy diet, how we hydrate is equally important as what we eat. By keeping in mind some of the essential hydration rules of Ayurveda, you can benefit from healthier digestion, softer skin, increased energy, and overall wellness. Improper hydration can lead to sluggish digestion, slowed metabolism, toxic accumulation, dryness or water retention, and general feelings of heaviness.

Here are the main principles to remember regarding daily water intake:

1. **Drink for your body type.** Kapha types should drink 5 to 6 cups of plain water daily; Pitta types, 6 to 7 cups daily; and Vata types, 8 to 10 cups daily.
2. **Begin your day with a cup of hot water.** This simple practice hydrates your system, awakens your vital organs, increases your digestion, flushes toxins, and aids in promoting elimination each morning.
3. **Never drink iced beverages.** This common habit will weaken digestion, slow your metabolism, constrict your gastrointestinal (GI) tract, and constrict circulation (causing cold hands and feet, etc.).
4. **Sip on warm water between meals.** Sipping on warm water between meals helps hydrate and detoxify your body steadily throughout the day.
5. **Do not drink any liquids before, during, or after meals.** Drinking liquids with meals waters down your digestive enzymes and can lead to indigestion, slow metabolism, and increased toxicity.

## Cold, Hot, or Lukewarm?

Ayurveda recommends you avoid excessively cold or iced beverages because they douse your digestive fire. This, in turn, can create constriction in the GI tract and limit food and enzymes from flowing freely. Hot water, on the other hand, promotes free flowing movement in the digestive tract. Hot water liquifies any toxins and works to flush them out of your system with ease. Here's a helpful example: Have you ever tried to wash your dishes with cold water? It is not very effective, and any oil residue becomes thick, viscous, and impossible to clean. This is very similar to the process that happens in your body.

If you have an aversion to drinking plain, hot water, add a splash of lemon or lime for a bit of flavor. In the hotter months, drinking room temperature or lukewarm water is acceptable and still carries many health benefits. However, if you are able to drink hot or warm water regularly, it will boost your digestion, promote healthy elimination, and improve your circulation. Adopting this daily habit gives you a simple—yet powerful—way to enhance your overall health and wellness.

## Tonics and Teas

For a tasty Ayurvedic staple used to maintain health and treat disorders, try tonics and herbal teas. You can include digestive teas before or between meals, detox teas for cleanses, calming tonics before bed, and rejuvenating tonics to energize your system and minimize the effects of aging.

To add some herbal goodness into your daily routine, try these tridoshic teas and tonics:

◆ **CCF and Ginger Tea (page 54)**— An Ayurvedic essential for flushing out toxins

◆ **Digestion Tonic (page 51)**—A digestive aid and wonderful addition to any weight-loss program

◆ **Golden Milk (page 56)**—Perfect for calming your energy before bed and promoting sound sleep

### SMALL ADJUSTMENTS: MEALTIMES

**1.** Eat on a healthy meal schedule. Consistently eating at the proper times helps create balance in your digestion, energy levels, mind, and emotions.

**2.** Make lunch the biggest meal of the day. Midday is when your digestive fires burn the brightest and you will need lots of fuel to keep that energy going strong until the evening.

**3.** Make dinner the lightest meal of the day. Your digestion and metabolism naturally slow down around 6:00 p.m. each evening and continue to slow until morning. Eating large meals too late can cause indigestion, disturbed sleep, weight gain, and toxicity in the system.

**4.** Always eat sitting down and avoid eating while driving, working on the computer, talking on the phone, or watching TV. Make meals your meditation! Eating sitting down, with full awareness, is essential to properly digesting your food and avoiding overeating.

**5.** Take a short walk after meals. This allows space and movement in the GI tract and can improve digestion as a whole. This recommendation is especially beneficial after larger meals and later meals.

# Your Ayurvedic Kitchen

As you begin your journey into the world of Ayurvedic cooking, making small adjustments in your kitchen will help make these dietary changes more accessible. These steps will pave your pathway to cooking success.

### Trying New Foods

Before jumping into the recipes, you may need to stock up on some new key ingredients. Most of these ingredients can be found at your local supermarket or health food store. When all else fails, you can find them online (on Amazon or websites that specialize in health food and spices such as Thrive Market, Vitacost, My Organic Grocery, and Mountain Rose Herbs). Here is a quick list to get you started:

- **Cooking oils:** coconut, sesame, and/ or sunflower

- **Ghee:** this is butter with the milk solids removed

- **Grains and legumes:** mung dal (yellow split mung bean), red lentils, and quinoa

- **Rice:** basmati

- **Seeds and nuts:** chia, flax, hemp, and pumpkin seeds; almonds and cashews

- **Spices:** brown mustard seeds, cardamom, cinnamon, cumin seeds, fennel seeds, ginger (fresh and dried), and turmeric

- **Vegetables:** carrots, celery, cilantro, kale, scallions, and zucchini

Set yourself up for success: Think about how much more likely you are to cook if you already have all the ingredients. If you feel overwhelmed about which ingredients to begin with, let's look at what's best for your dosha.

### If You're Kapha, Try . . .

Kapha types benefit most with heating, stimulating foods and spices such as dried ginger, black pepper, cayenne pepper, fresh lemon, onion, garlic, and brown mustard seeds. Although Kapha types should use cooking oils sparingly, the best options are sunflower oil (due to its lighter nature), sesame oil (which is warming), and ghee (which is tridoshic). In general, Kapha types should favor lighter grain options such as quinoa, buckwheat, or millet and limit heavier ones such as rice and oats. When it comes to sweeteners, honey is great for reducing Kapha and should be used over any other option.

### If You're Pitta, Try . . .

Pitta types naturally thrive with cooling, soothing foods to reduce the excessive heat they are prone to. Some Pitta kitchen essentials include fresh cilantro, limes, fennel, coriander seeds, cardamom, cumin, and scallions. The best cooking oils are ghee, coconut oil, and sunflower oil, all of which are very cooling. Basmati rice soothes Pitta, and white quinoa and oats can also be beneficial. Honey and molasses are often too heating for Pitta types and therefore those individuals should choose maple syrup as a healthy natural sweetener.

### If You're Vata, Try . . .

Vata types do best with warming, heavy, and oily foods to promote calm and reduce the cold, dry qualities that these body types often experience. Some Vata-reducing kitchen essentials include tahini, lemon, cinnamon, turmeric, ginger, brown mustard seeds, cumin, black pepper, nutmeg, mineral salt, garlic, and scallions. Vata types should use healthy oils generously, with the best oil options being sesame oil, almond oil, and ghee. Whole grains are very beneficial for grounding Vata, with basmati rice, white quinoa, and oats being some of the best. Vata does great with most natural sweeteners; molasses and honey are very warming and nutritious options.

## Keeping Things Spicy

One of the main principles of Ayurvedic cooking is spice, spice—and more spice! Spices not only add a decadent aroma, delicious flavor, and beautiful presence to your meals, but they possess a bounty of health benefits, too. All the spices used in this book are considered excellent digestive aids and will help you break down meals, absorb nutrients more efficiently, reduce gas and bloating, and promote healthy metabolism and elimination. Of these, ginger and turmeric are used the most, because they contain healing properties that aid in reducing inflammation, increasing immunity, cleansing the blood and liver, and stimulating the mind.

Since there are a wide range of spices in this book, it may be helpful to know which to focus on for your Ayurvedic constitution:

 **Kapha types**—Tend toward a slow metabolism and sleepiness after eating food, making heating and stimulating spices a must. Although *all* spices are beneficial for Kapha, the most beneficial include turmeric, dried ginger (best), fresh ginger, black pepper, cumin, clove, pink Himalayan salt (in moderation), and brown mustard seeds.

 **Pitta types**—Easily become overheated with too many hot spices. Therefore, Pitta types should favor cooling spices such as fennel, coriander, cumin, fresh ginger, cardamom, and turmeric and limit heating spices such as cayenne pepper, black pepper, sesame seeds, brown mustard seeds, salt, and ground ginger.

**Vata types**—Find much benefit by adding spices to their foods, because they tend to have irregular, weak digestion. Although most spices are great for Vata, the most healing are turmeric, fresh ginger (best), dried ginger, cumin, sesame seeds, brown mustard seeds, mineral salt, hing (asafetida), and fennel.

## A Flexible Approach

If you haven't noticed yet, Ayurveda has quite a few "food rules" to keep track of, which can make it feel overwhelming! Some of the more time-consuming dietary guidelines include always eat fresh meals, never eat leftovers, never use canned or frozen foods, limit eating out, avoid raw foods, and avoid prepackaged foods.

While following these guidelines will help you stay in balance and heal from a health condition, it's important to remain realistic to ensure you can keep up with your healthy diet without becoming resentful or burning out. Fortunately, in Ayurveda, there are always ways to make modifications to fit your needs.

When it comes to the dietary guidelines, remain flexible. For example, if your options are to either eat a home-cooked meal using canned beans or order a pizza, by all means opt for the canned beans. If you can either cook a large pot of oatmeal to eat throughout the week or eat cold cereal with milk every morning, then the reheated oatmeal is definitely the healthier option. If you love your raw smoothies and are not ready to part with them, then add some warming, digestive spices such as ginger, turmeric, and cinnamon to them.

In the end, it's important that you follow as many of these dietary guidelines as possible, but only while practicing self-compassion and keeping your expectations realistic. Cooking three fresh meals a day is not a viable option for most people, and you must arrive at a compromise that works for you.

### Saving Time

Although this diet may not be ideal in terms of eating 100 percent freshly prepared foods, you can save time by using some canned and frozen ingredients. Ultimately, you must be realistic and make healthy compromises to best meet your needs. With this in mind, using ready-made ingredients like canned chickpeas, store-bought hummus, or frozen vegetables once in a while can save you a lot of time and allow you to enjoy home-cooked meals during the week.

If you're ready to move away from canned goods and processed foods, another great time-saving tip is to make these ingredients yourself, and stock up for the week. For example, instead of using canned chickpeas, make a large batch of chickpeas to have on hand for the Chana Masala (page 146) or the Chickpea and Kale Brown Rice Bowl (page 150). Instead of store-bought hummus, make a large batch of Coconut Curry Hummus (page 98) to dress up your Summertime Salad (page 122) or Simply Delicious Lettuce Wrap (page 123).

### Leftovers

As previously mentioned, according to Ayurveda, leftovers are not great options. That's because they are considered to be devoid of Prana (life force), are lacking in nutrients, and can increase Vata with excessive consumption. Although this holds some truth, this isn't an all-or-nothing matter. If your choice is between eating leftovers for lunch or fast food, I think you can guess the healthier option. Think: progress not perfection!

When cooking with leftovers in mind, make enough for one or two extra days. Some reheating tips include:

- adding a splash of water to reduce any dryness
- reheating at a very low temperature
- stirring frequently to avoid burning
- adding in ghee and spices to liven up any dullness
- avoiding reheating your food more than once

## Keeping Things Simple

As you move forward on your journey toward a healthier lifestyle filled with fresh, homemade meals, try to keep things as simple as possible to avoid feeling overwhelmed or giving up completely. To that end, here's a simple seasonal plan that takes a lot of the guesswork out of meal-planning.

### Easy Seasonal Eating

| Winter | Spring | Summer | Fall |
|--------|--------|--------|------|
| Kapha Morning Tonic (page 48) | Detox Tonic (page 52) | Pitta Morning Tonic (page 49) | Vata Morning Tonic (page 50) |
| Masala Chai (page 55) | Kapha-Reducing Smoothie (page 62) | Hydrating Electrolyte Water (page 58) | Golden Milk (page 56) |
| Immunity Tonic (page 53) | Springtime Breakfast Scramble (page 88) | Tridoshic Summertime Smoothie (page 65) | Vata-Reducing Smoothie (page 64) |
| Golden Energy Buckwheat Breakfast (page 81) | Simply Spiced Quinoa Porridge (page 77) | Quick and Easy Overnight Oats (page 76) | Ojas-Increasing Oatmeal (page 74) |
| Kapha-Reducing Millet Porridge (page 82) | Curried Coconut and Veggie Soup (page 125) | Summertime Salad (page 122) | Quinoa Breakfast Smoothie (page 80) |

| Winter | Spring | Summer | Fall |
|---|---|---|---|
| Curried Black-Eyed Peas and Greens (page 148) | Spicy Sesame Rice (page 114) | Colorful Quinoa Salad (page 120) | Classic Cleansing Kitchari (page 132) |
| Kapha-Reducing Kitchari (page 134) | Spicy Red Lentil Dal (page 144) | Simply Delicious Lettuce Wrap (page 123) | Sweet Potato and Kale Quinoa Scramble (page 154) |
| Chana Masala (page 146) | Chickpea and Kale Brown Rice Bowl (page 150) | Tridoshic Quinoa and Veggie Stir-Fry (page 152) | Sautéed Kale and Golden Tahini Sauce (page 119) |
| Spinach Saag (page 116) | Roasted Zucchini Tahini Hummus (page 99) | Cucumber Raita (page 95) | Creamy Tahini Broth (page 100) |
| Winter-Spiced Rice Pudding (page 166) | Kapha-Reducing Kale Chips (page 102) | Ojas-Increasing Energy Balls (page 104) | Spiced Apples and Ghee (page 106) |

Now that you have a solid idea of how to adopt an appropriate Ayurvedic diet, let's dive into the specifics of how food choices can help you heal your body and mind.

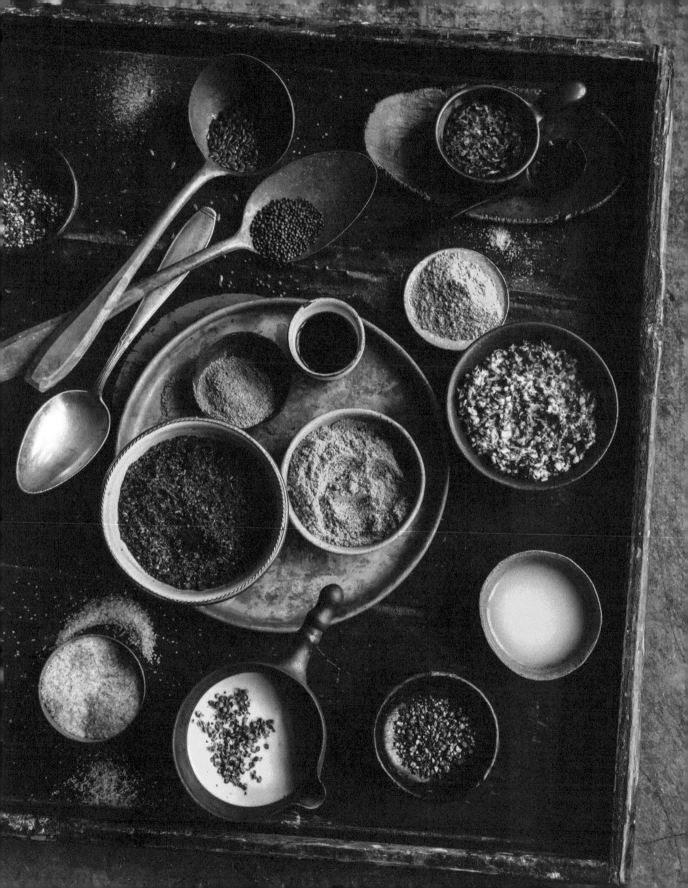

# EAT TO HEAL

There is an age-old saying: "With the proper diet, medicine is of no need; with an improper diet, medicine is of no use." This cannot be more true than in the eyes of Ayurveda, where your diet is a clear pathway to health—or disease. Food nourishes not only your physical body, but also your mind and consciousness. In this chapter, you will discover how food can heal, and learn about some basic remedies that can easily be made at home.

*Please note that these recommendations are not intended to cure any disease or replace your current medications. Always consult with your doctor before embarking on a new healing protocol.*

# Ayurveda and Disease

Ayurvedic medicine sees disease as a pathway paved over time through improper diet and lifestyle—a minor imbalance builds in strength, eventually resulting in disorder and disease. There are six stages to the disease process, known as *Samprapti.* By knowing in which stage you fall, you can see the severity of your condition as well as the level of effort you will need to put forth to rebuild your health.

Here is a quick overview of Samprapti.

STAGE 1–**Sanchaya:** In the first stage, the doshas become aggravated in their home bases: Kapha in the stomach, Pitta in the small intestine, and Vata in the colon. An example of this is gas and bloating caused by increased Vata.

STAGE 2–**Prakopa:** In this second stage, the doshas become further provoked due to an ongoing aggravation and begin to rise up from their home bases. To continue with our example, gas and bloating transform into indigestion, excessive burping, or pain in the back or chest due to continued Vata provocation.

STAGE 3–**Prasara:** In the third stage, the doshas have made their way into the bloodstream and spread throughout the body, seeking out a weak, vulnerable space to call home. Continuing with our example, this stage could cause dry skin, constricted circulation, numbness, ringing in the ears, or feelings of coldness from the ongoing Vata imbalance.

STAGE 4–**Sthana Samshraya:** In the fourth stage, the doshas begin to make a new home, moving into a place of weakness (e.g., a lifelong runner may have a weak space in their knees or hips). The imbalanced Vata will now move into areas such as the joints (causing cracking, popping, pain, and stiffness) or the mind (causing mild symptoms of sleep disturbance or restless mind).

STAGE 5–**Vyakti:** *Vyakti* means "manifest," and in this stage, mild symptoms experienced in stage 4 present as a marked disease. Joint issues progress to arthritis, and the Vata in the mind becomes chronic anxiety or insomnia.

STAGE 6–**Bhedha:** In stage 6, the disease that has manifested in stage 5 has been going on for so long, it creates further complications to the surrounding tissues and organs. The chronic Vata imbalance in the joints can cause bone loss and degeneration, and the ongoing anxiety or insomnia can lead to muscle wasting, nervous system disorders, weakness, or depletion.

By becoming in tune with our current state of well-being, we can understand when imbalance is happening and immediately treat the issue. It is much easier to treat a disorder in its earlier stages (ideally before stage 3). But don't become discouraged: No matter where you are, you can *always* improve your health by adopting appropriate diet and lifestyle practices.

## How Food Heals

Healthy food has the potential to heal your body, mind, and soul. Whether you are treating disease or maintaining health, proper food can nourish your being, bringing you optimal energy, mental-emotional balance, and an overall high quality of life.

### Healing Through Balance

The core of Ayurveda promotes achieving and maintaining physical, emotional, and spiritual balance. By maintaining health in these areas, you can move through life with ease, happiness, and contentment, avoiding illness and disease. Many of the disorders we sadly have come to see as normal signs of aging (diabetes, heart disease, arthritis, dementia, etc.) are far from this. By seeking balance, you can potentially steer away from these "inevitable" disorders and heal from any current conditions.

### Healing Through Prevention

Prevention presents the best path for healing. If your goal is prevention, this is the perfect book for your journey. In part II, you will discover multiple recipes that address specific areas of wellness. Whether you are looking to increase your bone health to avoid osteoporosis, lose weight to avoid metabolic disorders, or detoxify your body to increase energy, mental clarity, and digestive health, you'll have a wide variety of recipe options to make your effort a success!

# Healing Foods

Your food choices have unlimited potential when it comes to healing your body and mind. Although any imbalance will benefit from the proper food types, let's look at some of the more common conditions and the food options for healing them. You'll find this list is endless as you begin to discover the vast healing powers of Mother Nature! Please keep in mind, however, you should always consult with your doctor when experiencing any health issues.

## Tridoshic Foods for Healing

| Food | Health Benefits | How to Enjoy |
|------|-----------------|--------------|
| ALMONDS | High in fiber, protein, vitamin E, magnesium, and antioxidants; brightens complexion; promotes heart health; increases energy; builds strength | Almond milk, almond butter, smoothies, stir-fries, or simply by the handful |
| GHEE | Enhances energy and libido; promotes digestion and absorption; supports brain health; reduces inflammation | Add to any dish such as kitchari, soup, stir-fries, and oatmeal; use to replace cooking oil in any recipe |
| MUNG DAL | Easy to digest; detoxifies; energizes; high in protein, fiber, iron, calcium, folate, zinc, vitamin B, and antioxidants; great for weight loss | Eat as daily breakfast, lunch, or dinner; eat during times of illness, cleansing, or digestive disturbances |
| QUINOA | Complete protein source; high in fiber, iron, lysine, magnesium, and vitamin B; energizes and strengthens; aids in weight-loss programs | Salads, soups, porridges, smoothies, kitchari, sautés, stir-fries, and with steamed veggies |
| CILANTRO | Reduces heat, removes heavy metals, detoxifies, reduces inflammation | Garnish soups, stir-fries, kitchari, and stews; add to hummus, salads, salsa, or various dips; try Cilantro Juice (page 59). |

| Food | Health Benefits | How to Enjoy |
|------|-----------------|--------------|
| CUMIN | Increases digestion and absorption, burns toxins, reduces gas and bloating, relieves nausea, reduces menstrual cramps and uterine inflammation, increases lactation | Add to any savory recipe such as kitchari, stir-fries, and soups; try CCF and Ginger Tea (page 54) and Traditional Digestion Lassi (page 96) |
| TURMERIC | Reduces inflammation, strengthens and cleanses liver and blood, detoxifies, soothes asthma, heals skin and eye issues, helps prevent mental decline | Add to any recipe, including soups, stews, stir-fries, kitchari, dips, spreads, oatmeal, smoothies, drinks, and teas |
| GINGER | Improves digestion and absorption, reduces inflammation, detoxifies, increases immunity, alleviates asthma, stimulates the mind | Add to any recipe, including soups, stews, stir-fries, kitchari, dips, spreads, oatmeal, smoothies, drinks, and teas. |
| LIME | Stimulates digestion and metabolism, flushes toxins, makes food more digestible, provides a good source of vitamin C and antioxidants, boosts immunity | Add to any savory recipe such as kitchari, stir-fries, salads, hummus, and soups; try Pitta Morning Tonic (page 49) and Hydrating Electrolyte Water (page 58) |

# Eating for Digestion

Ayurveda says that the root of all disease stems from imbalanced digestive fire (known as *agni*) that governs all areas of your health—physical, mental, and emotional. This means that healing your digestive issues can bring about health in all other areas of your system.

Sluggish digestion caused by increased Kapha can lead to a dull appetite, sleepiness after eating, sadness, depression, brain fog, chronic fatigue, a buildup of toxins, weight gain, and metabolic disorders. Following a Kapha-reducing diet and lifestyle program will right the imbalance, increase your digestive fire, and, in turn, alleviate these common disorders.

High Pitta can lead to overactive digestive fire, triggering issues such as excessive heat, inflammation, loose stools, anger, judgment, frustration, hyperacidity, and skin disorders of all kinds. Following a Pitta-reducing diet and lifestyle program can help rebalance your system, soothe the overactive fire, and begin to heal these common conditions.

Weak, irregular digestive fire leads to anxiety, fear, worry, gas, bloating, constipation, insomnia, hyperactivity, restless mind, indecision, forgetfulness, and spaciness—all associated with increased Vata. Following a Vata-reducing diet and lifestyle can return you to a balanced state, strengthen your digestive fire, and alleviate the Vata disorder.

## Indigestion

Indigestion is a sign of a weak, sluggish digestive fire. You can be eating the healthiest food available, but if you are not breaking it down properly, that healthy food remains unprocessed and becomes toxic to your system.

Overall, your diet should remain light, simple, and easy to digest. Some essential foods to favor include mung dal, quinoa, buckwheat, millet, well-cooked vegetables, and soups. Using digestive spices such as ginger, turmeric, fennel, and black pepper will help increase digestive fire, as will lemon, lime, scallions, and ghee.

Here are some beneficial recipes for healing indigestion: Tridoshic Mung Dal and Quinoa Kitchari (page 140), Classic Cleansing Kitchari (page 132), Spicy Red Lentil Dal (page 144), Simply Steamed Veggies (page 124), and Golden Energy Buckwheat Breakfast (page 81). Drink Kapha Morning Tonic (page 48) each morning, and before lunch and dinner, and Digestion Tonic (page 51) between meals and before bed.

Improper food combinations, overeating, grazing, and excessive snacking are contraindicated. Always eat sitting down with full awareness, and avoid eating after 7:00 p.m. After eating, take a short walk; always avoid lying down after a meal.

## A Healing Cleanse

Ayurveda offers powerful and effective cleansing therapies. No matter the illness, this ancient science recommends you perform some level of detoxification before entering into a specific treatment to first establish a strong foundation. Ayurvedic cleansing programs are directed toward strengthening digestion, flushing out deep-rooted toxins, healing mental-emotional imbalance, treating disorder, and preventing disease.

The most common Ayurvedic at-home cleanse is the Kitchari Cleanse. This cleanse involves eating only kitchari for three to seven days, depending on your age, strength, state of health, and health care needs. During this time, you should avoid working, intense exercise, and all laborious activities, and focus on resting as much as possible. You are encouraged to also consume cleansing teas and herbs along with the kitchari to aid detoxification and produce stronger results such as improved energy, mental clarity, and a general sense of lightness. During the cleanse and for at least one week after, you must eliminate sugar, caffeine, and alcohol from your diet.

Although this cleanse benefits almost everyone, it's especially helpful for digestive issues, weight gain, slow metabolism, high blood pressure, high cholesterol, mental-emotional imbalances, diabetes, arthritis, skin disorders, autoimmune conditions, constipation, dry skin, low libido, infertility, and chronic fatigue.

Ideally, cleansing takes place in the fall and spring seasons because the weather is milder and these seasons represent a state of transition. I recommend cleansing at least once a year, modifying the level of intensity as needed. Keeping up with this type of program annually (or biannually) is an effective way to reset your digestion and mind—and system as a whole—to maintain balance throughout the rest of the year.

If you want to experience a Kitchari Cleanse, use the Classic Cleansing Kitchari (page 132) recipe as your base. With this mono-diet, I recommend drinking 1 cup of Detox Tonic (page 52) each morning, midday, and before bed, and drinking 1 cup of the CCF and Ginger Tea (page 54) 15 minutes before each meal. You can start drinking these tonics the week before you cleanse and continue with them several days after the cleanse ends to ensure a smooth transition.

When performed properly, the Kitchari Cleanse provides a wealth of health benefits, but it can just as easily become harmful if proper measures are not taken. Always use full caution before, during, and after undertaking any type of cleansing program.

As you decide the best time to do your Kitchari Cleanse, keep a few essential factors in mind. Here are some indications that it may *not* be the ideal time for you to cleanse:

- During the intense heat of summer or cold of winter
- Directly before, after, or during travel
- While going through any major life changes such as divorce, loss of a loved one, moving, or changing jobs
- During menstruation
- During pregnancy or the postpartum period
- While breastfeeding
- During times of heavy workload

Once you lay a solid foundation to begin the cleanse, it is important to ease your way into it by keeping your diet healthy and simple the week prior. Begin to include daily detoxifying teas and tonics to flush your system and prep your body. The post-cleansing period is extremely vital to establish your smooth transition into eating other foods and becoming more active. Keep your diet simple, focusing on well-cooked, light, easy-to-digest meals such as those detailed in the kitchari, dal, soup, and stir-fry recipes. Avoid all raw food, caffeine, alcohol, processed foods, and refined sugar for at least seven days post-cleanse. Slowly increase your workload and activity level over time, using awareness to honor your needs throughout your shift back into a normal routine.

# Ayurvedic Food Chart for Your Dosha

Before we move into the recipe section of this book, quickly review the doshic food chart provided. This chart will help you determine the most appropriate foods for your body type. Becoming familiar with the foods that calm your dosha is a great place to begin when adopting an Ayurvedic diet.

**If you are dual-doshic,** focus on foods and recipes that are balancing for both doshas, or those that align with the current season.

**If you are predominant in one dosha,** but your imbalance lies in another, honor the dosha in which the imbalance lies while taking good care to not push your main dosha out of balance. If possible, it's best to favor foods that are beneficial for both. For example, if you are Kapha, but currently have high Vata, you'll want to consume foods that reduce Vata without increasing Kapha, such as ghee, sesame oil, warming spices, honey, buckwheat, quinoa, and mung dal. When all else fails, focusing on tridoshic recipes is a foolproof way to maintain balance for all bodies in all seasons.

## Ayurvedic Food Chart

| Food Types | Best Foods for Kapha | Best Foods for Pitta | Best Foods for Vata |
|---|---|---|---|
| FRUIT | Apples, apricots, berries, cherries, cranberries, dry figs, grapes, lemons, limes, peaches, pears, pomegranate, prunes | Apples, avocado, sweet berries, sweet cherries, coconut, dates, figs, grapes, limes, ripe mango, peaches, pears, plums, pomegranate, raisins, watermelon | Apricots, avocado, bananas, berries, cherries, coconut, cooked apples, dates, fresh figs, grapes, lemons, limes, mangos, melons, oranges, papaya, peaches, pineapple, plums, soaked prunes, soaked raisins |

*continued on next page*

| Food Types | Best Foods for Kapha | Best Foods for Pitta | Best Foods for Vata |
|---|---|---|---|
| VEGETABLES | Asparagus, beets, broccoli, cabbage, carrots, cauliflower, celery, cilantro, corn, garlic, green beans, leafy greens, mushrooms, onions, parsley, peas, peppers, radishes, spinach, summer squash, tomatoes (cooked) | Asparagus, cooked beets, bitter melon, broccoli, cabbage, cauliflower, celery, cilantro, cucumber, green beans, leafy greens, mushrooms, parsley, winter and summer squash, sweet potatoes, white potatoes | Asparagus, beets, carrots, cilantro, cucumber, green beans, black olives, peas, spinach, winter and summer squash, sweet potato |
| GRAINS | Barley, buckwheat, corn, granola, millet, dry oats, quinoa, rye | Barley, basmati rice, buckwheat, granola, cooked oats, pasta, quinoa, whole wheat | Cooked oats, quinoa, rice, whole wheat |
| LEGUMES | Black beans, black-eyed peas, chickpeas, lentils, mung dal, pinto beans, split peas | Black beans, black-eyed peas, chickpeas, kidney beans, mung dal, pinto beans, split peas | Mung dal, red lentils |
| NUTS AND SEEDS | Almonds, chia seeds, flaxseed, popcorn (no salt or butter), pumpkin seeds, sunflower seeds | Almonds (soaked and peeled), chia seeds, coconut, flaxseed, popcorn, pumpkin seeds, sunflower seeds | Almonds, cashews, coconut, pecans, pistachios, walnuts, pumpkin seeds, sesame seeds, sunflower seeds, tahini |

| Food Types | Best Foods for Kapha | Best Foods for Pitta | Best Foods for Vata |
|---|---|---|---|
| FATS AND OILS | Almond, canola, corn, ghee, sesame (in moderation), sunflower | Avocado, coconut, flaxseed, ghee, olive, sunflower | Avocado, ghee, olive, sesame |
| DAIRY | Cottage cheese, ghee, goat cheese, goat milk | Milk, butter, ghee, goat cheese, sweet cream | Milk, butter, cheese, ghee, yogurt |
| MEAT AND FISH | Chicken (white), egg whites, fresh water fish, shrimp, turkey (white) | Chicken (white), egg whites, fresh water fish, turkey (white) | Beef, chicken, eggs, fish, salmon, shrimp, tuna, turkey (dark) |
| SPICES | Black pepper, brown mustard seeds, cardamom, cayenne, cinnamon, cloves, coriander, cumin, fennel, dry ginger, nutmeg, turmeric | Fresh basil, cardamom, cloves, coriander, cumin, fennel, fresh ginger, mint, parsley, turmeric | Black pepper, brown mustard seeds, cardamom, cinnamon, cloves, coriander, cumin, fennel, fresh ginger, hing (asafetida), nutmeg, turmeric |
| SWEETENERS | Fruit, honey, molasses | Cane sugar, coconut sugar, date sugar, fruit, maple syrup | Coconut sugar, date sugar, fruit, honey, maple syrup, molasses |

In part II, you will find a wide variety of healing recipes. You will discover everything from Ayurvedic drinks, teas, smoothies, and tonics to snacks, appetizers, main courses, and desserts. Some recipes you will notice represent more traditional Indian dishes such as the saag, chapati, raita, and various kitchari recipes, while others are more Westernized such as the stir-fries, smoothies, muffins, and kale chips. One common denominator is that all these recipes are made using only whole food ingredients, lots of digestive spices, and healthy, healing fats. All will help you see how to use food as medicine without compromising taste—or satisfaction.

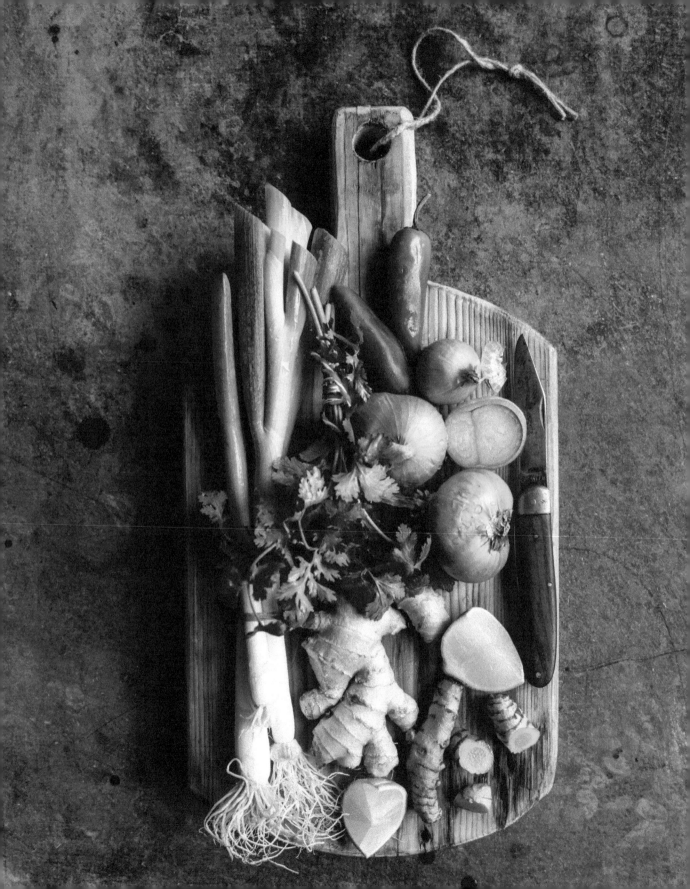

# PART II
## Recipes for Healing, Health, and Wellness

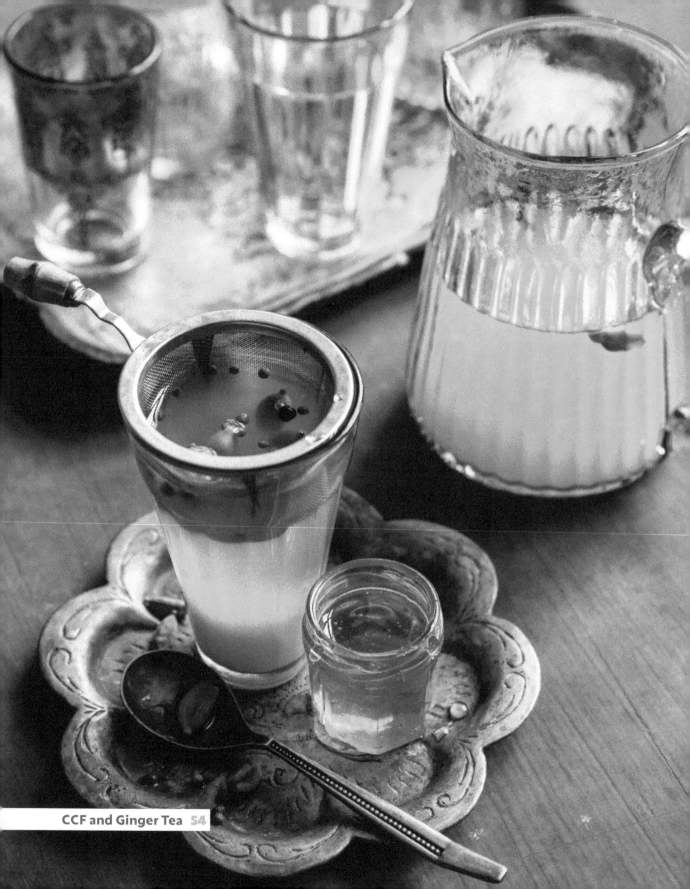

CCF and Ginger Tea **54**

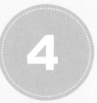

# DRINKS, TEAS, AND TONICS

# Kapha Morning Tonic

**GOOD FOR:** Weight Loss, Digestion, Metabolism, Detox, Congestion, Hydration, Immunity

**MAKES 1½ CUPS / PREP TIME: 5 MINUTES**

Enjoy this in the morning and begin your day with energy and vitality! This cleansing tonic is for Kaphas or anyone looking to lose weight or detoxify. When consumed during a time of illness, it can help ease a cold, fever, or flu, and remove congestion in the respiratory tract.

12 ounces hot water

Juice of ½ lemon

½ teaspoon apple cider vinegar

¼ to ½ teaspoon ground ginger

⅛ teaspoon freshly ground black pepper

2 teaspoons honey

1. Pour the hot water into a mug.

2. Add the lemon juice, apple cider vinegar, ginger, and black pepper. Stir well.

3. Allow the drink to cool slightly. Once it is at a drinkable temperature, stir in the honey.

4. Enjoy this drink first thing each morning on an empty stomach.

**+ HEALTH TIP:**

*Drink this tonic 30 minutes before each meal to aid in weight loss, sluggish digestion, and slow metabolism.*

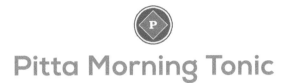

# Pitta Morning Tonic

**GOOD FOR:** Energy, Detox, Liver Health, Digestion, Hydration, Hyperacidity, Skin Disorders, Complexion, Inflammation

**MAKES 1½ CUPS / PREP TIME: 5 MINUTES**

This simple recipe includes a handful of ingredients that flush out toxins, alkalize the body, reduce inflammation, improve digestion, and beautify the complexion. This drink can also help strengthen, cleanse, and cool the liver. This morning tonic naturally brings you energy, hydration, and a strong foundation for your day to come!

12 ounces hot water

⅛ teaspoon cardamom powder

⅛ teaspoon turmeric powder

Juice of ½ lime

1 tablespoon aloe juice

2 to 3 teaspoons maple syrup

⅛ teaspoon baking soda

1. Pour the hot water into a mug.

2. Add the cardamom, turmeric, lime juice, aloe juice, and maple syrup. Stir well.

3. Mix in the baking soda right before drinking. This creates a lovely effervescence.

4. Enjoy this tonic first thing each morning on an empty stomach.

## + HEALTH TIP:

*To use this drink as a liver tonic, drink it each morning on an empty stomach, between breakfast and lunch, and again between lunch and dinner.*

# Vata Morning Tonic

**GOOD FOR:** Energy, Detox, Bone Health, Hydration, Constipation, Digestion, Anemia, Anxiety, Sleep Disorders, Pregnancy, Postpartum, Lactation

**MAKES 1½ CUPS / PREP TIME: 5 MINUTES**

This morning tonic is a wonderful way for Vata types to start each day. The ghee gently flushes toxins, strengthens the digestion, improves absorption, and promotes healthy elimination. The ashwagandha powder increases energy levels in the daytime, promotes sound sleep in the evening, reduces anxiety, and calms a restless mind.

12 ounces hot water

1 teaspoon molasses

¼ teaspoon ground ginger

½ teaspoon ashwagandha powder (optional, but recommended)

½ teaspoon ghee

1 teaspoon honey

1. Pour the hot water into a mug.

2. Add the molasses, ginger, ashwagandha (if using), and ghee. Stir well.

3. Allow the drink to cool slightly. Once it is at a drinkable temperature, stir in the honey.

4. Enjoy this tonic first thing each morning on an empty stomach.

**+ HEALTH TIP:**

*To alleviate insomnia symptoms, replace the hot water with warm milk (dairy is best, but almond milk is the next best) and drink 30 minutes before bed.*

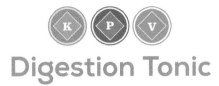

# Digestion Tonic

**GOOD FOR:** Digestion, Metabolism, Gas, Indigestion, Bloating, Weight Loss, Constipation, Detox, Energy, Immunity

**MAKES 6 CUPS / PREP TIME: 10 MINUTES / COOK TIME: 15 TO 20 MINUTES**

Healthy digestion is essential for treating and preventing all disease. It governs your mood, energy levels, and overall state of wellness. This powerful recipe helps increase your digestive fire and bring your body back to balance.

6 cups water

3 tablespoons finely minced fresh ginger (use 2 tablespoons for Pitta)

1 teaspoon coriander seeds, whole

1 teaspoon fennel seeds, whole

¼ teaspoon black peppercorns, whole (use ⅛ teaspoon for Pitta)

½ teaspoon hulled cardamom seeds, whole

¼ teaspoon turmeric powder

Juice of ½ lemon (use lime for Pitta)

1 to 2 teaspoons honey per serving

1. In a medium saucepan, bring the water and ginger to a boil, then reduce to a simmer.

2. Place the coriander, fennel, black peppercorns, and cardamom in a spice grinder or blender. Grind them until they have become a coarse powder.

3. Add the freshly ground spices and turmeric to the saucepan. Stir well.

4. Steep, mostly covered, while simmering for 15 to 20 minutes.

5. Strain the liquid into a large vessel for pouring. Stir in the lemon juice.

6. Pour the infusion into a mug. Allow it to cool slightly and then add in 1 to 2 teaspoons of honey per 8-ounce cup.

7. Drink 1 to 3 cups of the digestion tonic between meals daily.

8. Store in an airtight jar in the refrigerator for up to 5 days.

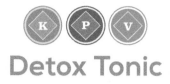

# Detox Tonic

**GOOD FOR:** Detox, Digestion, Illness, Metabolism, Weight Loss, Circulation

**MAKES 8 CUPS / PREP TIME: 10 MINUTES / COOK TIME: 20 MINUTES**

This spicy blend complements any cleanse. It flushes toxins, increases digestive fire, and promotes sweating. Only make this when detoxification is needed, such when you are experiencing illness, weak digestion, or a slow metabolism.

8 cups water

1 large beet, cubed
(1½ to 2 cups, chopped)

5 celery stalks, chopped

4 garlic cloves, thinly sliced
(use 2 cloves for Pitta)

1 cup cilantro, chopped

1 cup parsley, chopped

3 to 4 tablespoons finely minced
fresh ginger

1½ teaspoons black peppercorns,
whole (use ½ teaspoon for Pitta)

1 teaspoon fennel seeds, whole

Juice of 1 lemon (use lime for Pitta)

2 tablespoons olive oil

2 tablespoons apple cider vinegar
(use 1 tablespoon for Pitta)

1. Pour the water into a large stockpot. Add the beet, celery, garlic, cilantro, parsley, and ginger, cover, and bring to a boil.

2. Place the black peppercorns and fennel into a spice grinder or blender. Grind them to a powder and add them to the pot.

3. Reduce the heat to medium-low. Steep, covered, while simmering for at least 20 minutes.

4. Strain the liquid using a fine-mesh strainer.

5. Stir in the lemon juice, olive oil, and apple cider vinegar.

6. Serve warm. Drink 2 or 3 times daily during times of detoxification.

7. Store any extra in an airtight jar in the refrigerator for up to 5 days.

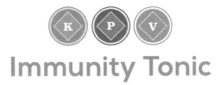

# Immunity Tonic

**GOOD FOR:** Congestion, Immunity, Nausea, Detox, Digestion, Metabolism, Weight Loss, Circulation, Inflammation, Arthritis

**MAKES 6 CUPS / PREP TIME: 10 MINUTES / COOK TIME: 20 MINUTES**

Drinking this infusion at the first onset of symptoms will help you prevent and treat illness. This spicy concoction boosts your immunity, increases your digestive fire, and promotes circulation.

6 cups water

1 tablespoon finely minced fresh ginger

2 large garlic cloves, finely minced

1 teaspoon minced jalapeño pepper

1 teaspoon turmeric powder

Juice of 1 lemon

6 teaspoons honey, divided

1. Pour the water into a large saucepan, cover, and bring to a boil.

2. Add the ginger, garlic, jalapeño pepper, and turmeric to the boiling water.

3. Reduce the heat to medium-low. Steep, mostly covered, while simmering for 20 minutes.

4. Strain the liquid using a fine-mesh strainer.

5. Stir in the lemon juice.

6. Pour the infusion into a mug. Allow it to cool slightly and then add in 1 teaspoon of honey per 8-ounce cup.

7. Drink every 2 to 3 hours during times of illness. Store in an airtight jar in the refrigerator for up to 5 days.

**+ HEALTH TIP:**

*This versatile tonic can also be used during times of cleansing, when you are trying to lose weight, or in the case of general Kapha imbalance.*

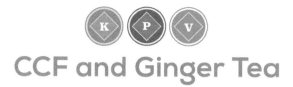

# CCF and Ginger Tea

**GOOD FOR:** Digestion, Detox, Gas, Bloating, Hyperacidity, Nausea, Malabsorption, Weight Loss, UTI, Allergies, Inflammation, Immunity, PMS, Pregnancy, Morning Sickness, Postpartum, Lactation

**MAKES 4 CUPS / PREP TIME: 5 MINUTES / COOK TIME: 15 TO 25 MINUTES**

A powerful digestive remedy, this savory blend is gentle enough for all body types. It's typically consumed between meals to flush toxins and reduce indigestion. This recipe is helpful to remedy cold, fever, flu, allergies, UTI, PMS, and morning sickness. If you're using this during a detoxification program or weight-loss regimen, drink 2 to 3 cups daily between meals.

4 cups water

1 tablespoon coriander seeds, whole

1 tablespoon cumin seeds, whole

1 tablespoon fennel seeds, whole

2 teaspoons finely minced fresh ginger

1. Pour the water into a medium saucepan, cover, and bring to a boil.

2. Once the water is boiling, reduce to a simmer and add the coriander, cumin, fennel, and ginger.

3. Simmer, mostly covered, for 15 to 25 minutes.

4. Strain the liquid using a fine-mesh strainer.

5. Serve warm. Drink at least 1 cup each day either between or before meals. For more severe digestive issues, drink 3 cups daily.

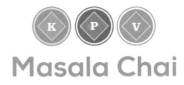

# Masala Chai

**GOOD FOR:** Energy, Digestion, Circulation, Bone Health

**MAKES 4 CUPS / PREP TIME: 5 MINUTES / COOK TIME: 20 MINUTES**

Starting the day with this sweet and spicy chai makes for a beautiful ritual! Although there is some caffeine in the black tea, the cardamom, cinnamon, and ginger calm the adrenals and allow your body to process the caffeine better, providing you with balanced, sustainable energy.

2 cups whole milk or Tridoshic Almond Milk (page 57, use almond milk for Kapha)

2 cups water

2 tablespoons finely minced fresh ginger

2 cinnamon sticks

8 teaspoons loose-leaf black tea (or 8 tea bags)

¼ teaspoon hulled cardamom seeds, whole

¼ teaspoon black peppercorns, whole

10 to 12 cloves, whole

1 to 2 teaspoons honey per cup (optional)

1. Pour the milk and water into a medium saucepan, cover, and heat to just below a boil.

2. Reduce the heat to a simmer and add the ginger, cinnamon sticks, and black tea.

3. Coarsely grind the cardamom, peppercorns, and cloves in a spice grinder or blender. Add the ground spices to the pan.

4. Steep, mostly covered, on simmer for 15 to 20 minutes. Stir every 5 minutes.

5. Strain the liquid and serve. Cool slightly and add 1 to 2 teaspoons of honey (if using) per 8-ounce serving. Store any extra in an airtight jar in the refrigerator for up to 3 or 4 days.

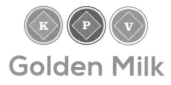

# Golden Milk

**GOOD FOR:** Anxiety, Sleep Disorders, Depression, Focus, Circulation, Inflammation, Arthritis, Bone Health, Nervous System Health, Anemia, Complexion

**MAKES 1 CUP / COOK TIME: 20 MINUTES**

Golden Milk is a great evening tonic for nourishing Kapha, soothing Pitta, and calming Vata. This deliciously creamy drink is often used to quiet the mind, boost the mood, promote sound sleep, strengthen the bones, reduce inflammation, and beautify the complexion. With its amazing taste and long list of health benefits, Golden Milk will soon become a regular part of your nighttime routine.

1 cup whole milk or Tridoshic Almond Milk

½ cup water

½ teaspoon turmeric powder

½ teaspoon ashwagandha powder (optional)

¼ teaspoon ground ginger

⅛ teaspoon cardamom powder

Pinch freshly ground black pepper

1 cinnamon stick

3 saffron threads

½ teaspoon ghee (omit for Kapha)

1 teaspoon honey

1. In a small saucepan, heat the milk and water to just below a boil, and then reduce to a simmer.

2. Add the turmeric, ashwagandha (if using), ginger, cardamom, black pepper, cinnamon stick, saffron, and ghee to the pan. Stir well until the powdered spices have dissolved.

3. Simmer, mostly covered, for 20 minutes, stirring every 5 minutes.

4. Pour the milk into a mug. Let it cool to a drinkable temperature and then stir in the honey.

5. Sip on this beverage up to 30 minutes before bed each night.

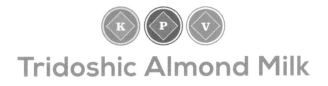

# Tridoshic Almond Milk

**GOOD FOR:** Energy, Immunity, Libido, Brain Health, Nervous System Health, Complexion

**MAKES 4 CUPS / PREP TIME: 15 MINUTES (PLUS 2 TO 4 HOURS SOAK TIME)**

Freshly made almond milk tastes much better than store-bought and is much healthier for you! This simple recipe requires only two ingredients: almonds and water. It is tridoshic and a great dairy alternative for Kaphas or anyone sensitive to dairy.

| | |
|---|---|
| 40 almonds | 4 cups water |

1. In a small bowl of water, soak the almonds for at least 2 to 4 hours to soften the skins.
2. Drain the almonds and discard the water.
3. Peel the almonds by squeezing each one with your index finger and thumb. This should allow easy removal and should take only a few minutes altogether.
4. Place 4 cups of water and the peeled almonds into a blender.
5. Blend on high for 3 to 5 minutes.
6. After the blending is complete, use cheesecloth or a fine-mesh strainer to strain the milk into a quart-size glass jar.
7. Store in an airtight jar and refrigerate for up to 3 or 4 days. Separation may occur. Shake the jar before each use.

**INGREDIENT TIP:**

*For a sweet almond milk, add 1 to 2 tablespoons of maple syrup for Vata and Pitta types, or 1 to 2 tablespoons of honey for Vata and Kapha types.*

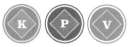

# Hydrating Electrolyte Water

**MAKES 4 CUPS / PREP TIME: 5 TO 10 MINUTES**

Here is a summertime essential for staying cool, hydrated, and ener-gized. In times of dehydration, excessive heat, heavy sweating, intense exercise, and illness, your body can become depleted of natural energy sources, causing muscle weakness and fatigue. This simple drink recipe refuels you, while cooling excessive heat in your body.

4 cups water

Juice of ½ lime

2 to 3 teaspoons maple syrup

Pinch mineral salt, pink Himalayan salt, or sea salt

10 to 15 fresh mint leaves (optional)

1. Fill a quart-size glass jar with room-temperature water.
2. Add the lime juice, maple syrup, and a pinch of salt.
3. Chop the fresh mint leaves (if using) and add them to the drink mixture.
4. Let the mint leaves steep for at least 15 minutes.
5. Cover the jar with an airtight lid and shake several times.
6. Strain out the mint leaves and serve.
7. Store in an airtight jar in the refrigerator for up to 5 days.

**INGREDIENT TIP:**

*For more cooling, hydrating properties, add sliced cucumber, a splash of raw coconut water, or a tablespoon of aloe juice.*

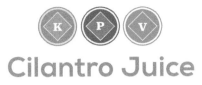

# Cilantro Juice

**GOOD FOR:** Complexion, Inflammation, Allergies, Liver Health, Kidney Health, UTI, Excessive Heat, Hot Flashes

**MAKES 4 CUPS / PREP TIME: 10 MINUTES**

Refreshing with a mild, pleasant taste, Cilantro Juice is a tridoshic home remedy for cooling excessive heat and reducing high Pitta. It provides gentle detoxification and is known to remove heavy metals from your tissues. It is often used for treating eczema, psoriasis, acne, rash, and itchy skin. As a natural anti-inflammatory, antihistamine source, it can be used for relief throughout allergy season.

1 bunch of cilantro                    4 cups water

1. Wash the cilantro thoroughly, removing any dirt. Chop the cilantro, using the stems and leaves.
2. Place the water in a blender and then add the cilantro.
3. Blend on high for 2 to 4 minutes. There should be no chunks leftover, only a fine pulp.
4. Strain any remaining pulp using a fine-mesh strainer or a cheesecloth.
5. Drink 1 cup of cilantro juice 1 to 3 times a day. Store in the refrigerator for up to 4 days.

**+ HEALTH TIP:**
*Use the leftover pulp to apply to your skin for treating rash, itchiness, psoriasis, eczema, or any skin disorder.*

Carrot-Beet Bliss Smoothie, Papaya Apricot Chia Seed Smoothie, and Rejuvenating Almond-Date Shake   67, 68, and 70

# SMOOTHIES

# Kapha-Reducing Smoothie

**GOOD FOR:** Energy, Digestion, Heart Health, Skin Health, Hair Health, Brain Health, High Cholesterol, High Blood Pressure

**MAKES 2 CUPS / PREP TIME: 10 MINUTES**

This Kapha-reducing smoothie is made with light, low-sugar fruits, an unsweetened liquid base, and a large amount of warming digestive spices. The antioxidant-rich cacao energizes, and counteracts any Kapha sluggishness. The hemp seeds and flaxseed give this smoothie a bit more creaminess and provide you with heart-healthy, brain-boosting omega-3s.

1 cup Tridoshic Almond Milk (page 57)

1 cup strawberries

1 cup raspberries

½ apple, chopped (about ¾ cup)

1 tablespoon hemp seeds

1 tablespoon flaxseed

1 tablespoon cacao powder

1 teaspoon ground cinnamon

½ teaspoon ground ginger

⅛ teaspoon turmeric powder

1 teaspoon honey

**1.** Put the almond milk, strawberries, raspberries, apple, hemp seeds, flaxseed, cacao, cinnamon, ginger, turmeric, and honey into a blender.

**2.** Blend on high for 2 to 3 minutes or until a completely smooth texture has been reached.

**3.** Enjoy this smoothie as an energizing breakfast or a midday boost during the late spring and summer seasons.

**+ HEALTH TIP:**

*Try doubling the ginger power and adding 5 black peppercorns for even greater Kapha-reducing, metabolism-boosting results.*

# Pitta-Reducing Smoothie

**GOOD FOR:** Energy, Digestion, Hydration, Electrolyte Balance, Excessive Heat, Heart Health, Skin Health, Hair Health, Eye Health, Liver Health, Immunity

**MAKES 2 CUPS / PREP TIME: 15 MINUTES**

This cooling, Pitta-soothing smoothie recipe is a delicious way to make it through hot summer days. It boosts energy, increases digestion, and replenishes essential electrolyte balance. The avocado, aloe, lime, cardamom, turmeric, and rose petals are added to reduce inflammation, calm agitation, tone the liver, and balance out your Pitta all summer long. You can order rose petals online at Mountain Rose Herbs or find them at your local herb shop.

1 cup coconut water

4 fresh figs

1 small sweet, ripe mango, peeled and chopped

½ avocado

Fresh ginger (1-inch cube), minced

Juice of ¼ lime

2 tablespoons aloe juice

1 tablespoon dried rose petals

⅛ teaspoon cardamom powder

⅛ teaspoon turmeric powder

1. Put the coconut water, figs, mango, avocado, ginger, lime juice, aloe juice, rose petals, cardamom, and turmeric into a blender.

2. Blend on high for 2 to 3 minutes or until a completely smooth texture has been reached.

3. Enjoy this smoothie as an energizing breakfast, a midday pick-me-up, or post-workout rejuvenator during the late spring and summer seasons.

# Vata-Reducing Smoothie

**GOOD FOR:** Digestion, Constipation, Energy, Immunity, Anxiety, Complexion, Eye Health, Brain Health, Heart Health

**MAKES 2 CUPS / PREP TIME: 5 MINUTES / COOK TIME: 10 TO 15 MINUTES**

Here is a delicious, warming smoothie recipe to ground your energy anytime Vata is elevated. This smoothie is strengthening, energizing, and immune-boosting, and simultaneously soothing for your mind and nervous system.

1½ packed cups chopped sweet potato (½-inch cubes)

1 cup Tridoshic Almond Milk (page 57)

¼ cup plain yogurt

Fresh ginger (1-inch cube), minced

1 teaspoon ground cinnamon

⅛ teaspoon cardamom powder

⅛ teaspoon turmeric powder

3 saffron threads

½ teaspoon vanilla extract

2 to 3 teaspoons honey

1. Place a steamer basket in a medium saucepan. Fill the pan with water until it reaches just below the steamer basket. Bring the water to a boil.

2. Put the sweet potato in the basket and cover the pan. Cook on medium-low for 10 to 12 minutes or until the sweet potato is completely soft all the way through.

3. While steaming the sweet potato, put the almond milk, yogurt, ginger, cinnamon, cardamom, turmeric, saffron, vanilla, and honey in a blender.

4. Once the sweet potato is cooked, add it to the blender.

5. Blend on high for 2 to 4 minutes and serve.

6. Enjoy this warm smoothie recipe during the fall and winter seasons.

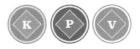

# Tridoshic Summertime Smoothie

**GOOD FOR:** Energy, Digestion, Excessive Heat, Heart Health, Brain Health, Skin Health, Liver Health, Inflammation

**MAKES 2 CUPS / PREP TIME: 10 MINUTES (PLUS 15 MINUTES TO SOAK)**

Here is a delightfully refreshing smoothie for the summer season that all can enjoy. It is very cooling for Pitta, light enough for Kapha, and contains healthy fats for Vata. Instead of containing a creamy or sweetened base, this tridoshic smoothie has hibiscus tea for added lightness, flavor, and extra healing power.

1 tablespoon chia seeds

1½ cups chilled hibiscus tea (use another herbal tea or water if unavailable)

1 cup strawberries

1 cup blueberries

1 small peach, chopped

1 avocado (use ½ for Kapha)

1 tablespoon dried rose petals

1 tablespoon hemp seeds

1 to 2 teaspoons honey (use maple syrup for Pitta)

1. In a cup, soak the chia seeds in the hibiscus tea (or herbal tea or water) for at least 15 minutes.

2. Pour the hibiscus tea and soaked chia seeds into a blender. Add the strawberries, blueberries, peach, avocado, rose petals, hemp seeds, and honey.

3. Blend on high for 2 to 3 minutes or until a completely smooth texture has been reached.

4. Enjoy this smoothie as a light breakfast or cooling snack throughout the summer.

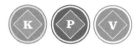

# Antioxidant Energy Smoothie

**GOOD FOR:** Energy, Immunity, Brain Health, Heart Health, Skin Health, Inflammation, Cancer Prevention

**MAKES 2 CUPS / PREP TIME: 10 MINUTES (PLUS 20 MINUTES TO SOAK)**

The Antioxidant Energy Smoothie wakes you up in the morning! It includes powerful antiaging, antioxidant-rich foods, including blueberries, goji berries, cacao, and spirulina. But the health benefits don't end there! Eating these well-known superfoods on a regular basis has been shown to uplift the mood, stimulate the brain, increase energy, and boost immunity.

2 tablespoons goji berries

1 cup Tridoshic Almond Milk (page 57)

½ banana (omit for Kapha)

1 cup blueberries

½ avocado (use ¼ for Kapha)

1 tablespoon hemp seeds

1 tablespoon sunflower seeds

1 tablespoon cacao powder (omit or use 1 teaspoon for Kapha)

1 teaspoon spirulina

3 saffron threads

1. In a cup, soak the goji berries in the almond milk for at least 20 minutes.

2. Pour the almond milk and soaked goji berries into a blender. Add the banana, blueberries, avocado, hemp seeds, sunflower seeds, cacao, spirulina, and saffron.

3. Blend on high for 2 to 3 minutes, or until a completely smooth texture has been reached.

4. Enjoy this smoothie as an energizing breakfast or a midday pick-me-up.

# Carrot-Beet Bliss Smoothie

**GOOD FOR:** Energy, Complexion, Constipation, Circulation, Anemia, Women's Health, Digestion, Liver Health, Heart Health, Muscle Recovery, Inflammation, Pregnancy, Postpartum

**MAKES 4 CUPS / PREP TIME: 15 MINUTES / COOK TIME: 10 MINUTES**

Here is a vibrant smoothie recipe that is as beautiful as it is delicious! Due to the nourishing, grounding nature of the ingredients, this is an ideal smoothie option for Vatas, and can even be enjoyed in the cooler seasons as long as it is served slightly warm.

1 large beet, chopped into small cubes (about 1½ cups)

1 medium carrot, sliced thin (about ½ cup)

2 cups Tridoshic Almond Milk (page 57)

½ avocado

Fresh ginger (1-inch cube), finely minced

1 teaspoon ground cinnamon

⅛ teaspoon cardamom powder

⅛ teaspoon turmeric powder

½ teaspoon vanilla extract

1 tablespoon honey

2 teaspoons maple syrup

1. Place a steamer basket in a medium saucepan. Fill the pan with water until it reaches just below the steamer basket. Bring the water to a boil.

2. Place the beets and carrots into the steamer basket. Steam, mostly covered, over medium-low heat for 8 to 10 minutes, or until the veggies are soft and well-cooked.

3. Put the steamed beets and carrots into a blender. Add the almond milk, avocado, ginger, cinnamon, cardamom, turmeric, vanilla, honey, and maple syrup.

4. Blend on high for 2 to 3 minutes, or until a smooth and creamy texture has been reached.

5. Enjoy this smoothie as an energizing breakfast, a healthy snack, or a muscle-healing, post-workout recovery aid.

# Papaya Apricot Chia Seed Smoothie

**GOOD FOR:** Digestion, Constipation, Inflammation, Immunity, Liver Health, Eye Health, Skin Health, Heart Health, Pregnancy, Postpartum

**MAKES 2 CUPS / PREP TIME: 10 MINUTES (PLUS 20 MINUTES TO SOAK)**

Give your digestion a boost with this flavorful papaya smoothie. Papaya contains enzymes that are beneficial for promoting healthy digestion and elimination. The apricot and chia seeds, when soaked, provide a wealth of fiber and lubricate the colon to lend a helping hand as well.

1 tablespoon chia seeds

7 dried apricots

1 cup water

2 cups chopped papaya

1 tablespoon minced fresh ginger

1 tablespoon shredded coconut

1 teaspoon coconut oil

1 teaspoon honey

**1.** Soak the chia seeds and dried apricots in a cup of water for at least 20 minutes.

**2.** Put the water, chia seeds, and apricots into a blender. Add the papaya, ginger, coconut, coconut oil, and honey.

**3.** Blend on high for 2 to 3 minutes, or until a completely smooth texture has been reached.

**4.** Enjoy this smoothie as a healthy breakfast.

# Probiotic Power Seed Drink

**GOOD FOR:** Strength, Energy, Rejuvenation, Digestion, Constipation, Skin Health, Hair Health, Heart Health, Bone Health, Pregnancy, Postpartum, Lactation

**MAKES 2 CUPS / PREP TIME: 10 MINUTES (PLUS 20 MINUTES TO SOAK)**

This probiotic drink is a delicious way to incorporate a variety of healing foods into one healthy snack. This nourishing recipe can be enjoyed up to 2 to 3 times a week for increasing strength, promoting rejuvenation, and balancing your Pitta and Vata.

---

1 tablespoon chia seeds

1¼ cup raw coconut water

½ cup plain yogurt

1 tablespoon hemp seeds

1 tablespoon raw pumpkin seeds

1 teaspoon finely minced fresh ginger

½ teaspoon ground cinnamon

⅛ teaspoon turmeric powder

⅛ teaspoon cardamom powder

1 teaspoon vanilla extract

2 to 3 teaspoons honey

---

1. Soak the chia seeds in the coconut water for at least 20 minutes.

2. Pour the chia seeds and coconut water into a blender. Add the yogurt, hemp seeds, pumpkin seeds, ginger, cinnamon, turmeric, cardamom, vanilla, and honey.

3. Blend on high for 2 to 3 minutes, or until a completely smooth and creamy texture has been reached.

4. Drink 8 ounces of this power drink as a nourishing breakfast shake or an energizing snack.

# Rejuvenating Almond-Date Shake

**GOOD FOR:** Energy, Rejuvenation, Vitality, Immunity, Complexion, Mood Enhancement, Age Prevention, Longevity, Pregnancy, Postpartum, Lactation

**MAKES 2 CUPS / PREP TIME: 20 MINUTES
(PLUS 2 TO 4 HOURS TO SOAK, OPTIONAL)**

This shake is a delicious variation on a classic Ayurvedic remedy. The almonds, dates, ghee, honey, rose petals, and saffron give this shake a rich, sweet flavor and are known to increase vitality (known as Ojas), boost the mood, beautify the complexion, prevent signs of aging, and enhance cellular rejuvenation.

15 almonds

2 medjool dates, pitted and soaked

1½ cups water

¼ teaspoon ground ginger

¼ teaspoon turmeric powder

⅛ teaspoon cardamom powder

1 tablespoon dried rose petals

3 saffron threads

½ teaspoon vanilla extract

1 teaspoon ghee

1 teaspoon honey

1. Soak the almonds in a cup of water for 2 to 4 hours (optional).

2. In 1½ cups of water, soak the pitted dates for at least 20 minutes. Reserve the liquid.

3. Drain the almonds and discard the water. Peel the almonds by squeezing each one with your index finger and thumb for easy removal.

4. Put the almonds, dates, and the date water into a blender.

5. Add the ginger, turmeric, cardamom, rose petals, saffron, vanilla, ghee, and honey to the blender.

6. Blend on high for 3 to 5 minutes, or until a completely smooth texture has been reached. If there are remaining chunks, strain the drink through a fine-mesh strainer.

7. Enjoy as an energizing breakfast or snack. (Due to its heavy and sweet nature, avoid drinking more than three times a week.)

# Chocolate Banana Date Shake

**GOOD FOR:** Energy, Vitality, Digestion, Constipation, Complexion, Mood Enhancement

**MAKES 2 CUPS / PREP TIME: 10 MINUTES (PLUS 20 MINUTES TO SOAK)**

This Chocolate Banana Date Shake is healthy enough to be enjoyed as a snack and delicious enough to be called a dessert. Because of the heavy, sweet nature of this drink, this recipe is not recommended for Kaphas or anyone with a Kapha imbalance.

---

3 or 4 medjool dates

1½ cups Tridoshic Almond Milk (page 57)

1 medium banana (use ½ banana for Pitta)

1 small avocado or ½ large avocado

1 tablespoon cacao powder (omit or use 1 teaspoon for Vata)

½ teaspoon vanilla extract

---

1. Soak the pitted dates in the almond milk for at least 20 minutes.

2. Pour the almond milk and dates into a blender. Add the banana, avocado, cacao, and vanilla.

3. Blend on high for 2 to 3 minutes, or until a completely smooth texture has been reached.

4. Enjoy occasionally as a decadent breakfast or an energizing snack. (Due to its heavy and sweet nature, avoid drinking more than once or twice a week.)

Golden Energy Buckwheat Breakfast  **81**

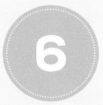

# BREAKFASTS

# Ojas-Increasing Oatmeal

**GOOD FOR:** Energy, Immunity, Libido, Muscle Strength, Heart Health, High Cholesterol, Inflammation, Pregnancy, Postpartum, Lactation

**SERVES 2 TO 3 / PREP TIME: 5 MINUTES / COOK TIME: 25 MINUTES**

Ojas is the biological energy that is responsible for our vitality, immunity, longevity, and glow. This dish is perfect for increasing essential Ojas in the body, calming the nervous system (Vata), and cooling off excessive heat (Pitta).

3¼ cups water

1 cup steel-cut oats

⅛ teaspoon salt

20 raisins

2 medjool dates, pitted and chopped

3 tablespoons shredded coconut, divided

1 tablespoon almond butter

1½ teaspoons ground cinnamon

½ teaspoon ground ginger

¼ teaspoon cardamom powder

1 teaspoon vanilla extract

2 teaspoons ghee

1 to 2 tablespoons honey (optional; use maple syrup for Pitta)

Dash ground cinnamon, for garnish

1. In a medium saucepan, bring the water to a boil. Reduce the heat to medium-low.

2. Add the oats and salt. Cook the oats, mostly covered, for 20 minutes. Stir every 7 to 10 minutes.

3. Turn the heat off but keep the pan on the hot burner. Add the raisins, dates, 2 tablespoons of coconut, almond butter, cinnamon, ginger, cardamom, vanilla, and ghee. Stir well. Cover and let sit for 5 minutes.

4. Serve into bowls and add 1 to 3 teaspoons of honey (if using), a dash of cinnamon, and a sprinkle of the remaining coconut to each serving.

5. Sit, eat, enjoy, and energize.

# Carrot Cake Oatmeal

**GOOD FOR:** Energy, Strength, Digestion, Eye Health, Heart Health, Skin Health, Brain Health, High Cholesterol, Inflammation, Pregnancy, Postpartum, Lactation

**SERVES 2 / PREP TIME: 5 MINUTES / COOK TIME: 25 MINUTES**

This recipe is as decadent as it sounds—and it's healthy, too! Adding carrots to your morning meal allows you to get a head start on your daily vegetable quota while offering a sweet taste and beautiful color to everyday oats. Pitta and Vata types can enjoy this throughout the fall and winter seasons.

3 cups water

1 cup steel-cut oats

1 cup grated carrots

Large pinch salt

2 cinnamon sticks

½ cup Tridoshic Almond Milk (page 57)

30 to 40 raisins

¼ cup walnut pieces

2 teaspoons ground cinnamon

¼ teaspoon cardamom powder

½ teaspoon ground ginger

¼ teaspoon turmeric powder

1 teaspoon vanilla extract

2 teaspoons ghee

2 to 4 teaspoons maple syrup

Ground cinnamon, for garnish

1. In a medium saucepan, bring the water to a boil. Reduce the heat to medium-low. Add the oats, carrots, salt, and cinnamon sticks.

2. Cook the oats, mostly covered, for 15 to 20 minutes. Stir every 5 minutes.

3. Turn the heat off but keep the pan on the hot burner. Add the almond milk, raisins, walnuts, cinnamon, cardamom, ginger, turmeric, vanilla, and ghee. Stir well. Cover and let sit for 5 minutes.

4. Serve into bowls and add 1 to 2 teaspoons of maple syrup and a dash of cinnamon to each serving.

5. Sit, share, and eat in good company.

## Quick and Easy Overnight Oats

**GOOD FOR:** Energy, Digestion, Constipation, Heart Health, Bone Health, High Cholesterol, Blood Sugar Balance, Pregnancy, Postpartum, Lactation

**SERVES 1 TO 2 / PREP TIME: 10 MINUTES (PLUS OVERNIGHT TO SOAK)**

This recipe allows you to prepare your breakfast in the evening and wake up to a hearty, nourishing meal. Since this oatmeal is typically eaten at room temperature (or cooler), it is best enjoyed during the spring and summer seasons.

1 cup Tridoshic Almond Milk (page 57), divided

¼ cup plain yogurt

½ teaspoon vanilla extract

2 teaspoons maple syrup

½ teaspoon cacao powder (omit for Vata)

½ teaspoon ground cinnamon

¼ teaspoon ground ginger

Pinch cardamom powder

2 medjool dates, pitted and finely chopped

½ cup rolled oats

4 tablespoons Morning Energy Mix (page 180), divided

1. Pour ¾ cup of almond milk into a glass jar with a lid.

2. Add the yogurt, vanilla, maple syrup, cacao, cinnamon, ginger, and cardamom and stir well.

3. Add the dates, oats, and 2 tablespoons of the Morning Energy Mix and stir well.

4. Cover the jar and refrigerate it until morning.

5. Take the oats out of the refrigerator at least 1 hour before eating to allow them to come to room temperature (Ayurveda discourages eating this meal cold). Vatas will benefit from slightly warming the oats by immersing the jar in hot water before eating.

6. Once you are ready to eat, stir in 1 to 2 tablespoons of the Morning Energy Mix. If the oats have become too thick, add the remaining ¼ cup of almond milk.

7. Eat, enjoy, and energize!

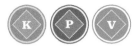

# Simply Spiced Quinoa Porridge

**GOOD FOR:** Energy, Digestion, Constipation, Weight Loss, Heart Health, Blood Sugar Balance, Pregnancy, Postpartum

**SERVES 2 / PREP TIME: 5 MINUTES / COOK TIME: 20 MINUTES**

The Simply Spiced Quinoa Porridge is a perfect breakfast recipe all year round. It is light enough for the spring and summer seasons, and warming enough for the fall and winter. Quinoa is a healthy grain choice for keeping all doshas in balance, making this a foolproof recipe for the whole family to enjoy.

2¼ cups water

1 cup quinoa

1 cinnamon stick

30 raisins

¾ cup Tridoshic Almond Milk (page 57)

2 teaspoons hemp seeds

2 teaspoons shredded coconut (omit for Kapha)

1 teaspoon ground cinnamon

½ teaspoon ground ginger

¼ teaspoon cardamom powder

1 teaspoon ghee

2 to 4 teaspoons honey

Dash ground cinnamon, for serving

1. In a medium saucepan, bring the water to a boil.

2. Reduce the heat to low, and add the quinoa and cinnamon stick. Cover and cook for 12 to 15 minutes.

3. Check the quinoa for doneness at 12 minutes. If more time is needed, continue to cook, checking every minute.

4. Once done, turn off the heat, but leave the pan on the warm burner. Add the raisins, almond milk, hemp seeds, coconut, cinnamon, ginger, cardamom, and ghee. Stir well and replace the cover, leaving the porridge to sit for 5 minutes more.

5. Serve the porridge. Once it has cooled slightly, add 1 to 2 teaspoons of honey per bowl. Sprinkle with cinnamon and add a splash of almond milk.

# Morning Energy Quinoa Porridge

**GOOD FOR:** Energy, Digestion, Constipation, Weight Loss, Heart Health, Blood Sugar Balance, Pregnancy, Postpartum

**SERVES 2 / PREP TIME: 5 MINUTES / COOK TIME: 15 MINUTES**

The heartiness of this quinoa porridge makes it ideal for the fall and winter seasons. The ground quinoa resembles cream of wheat in texture. Adding almond milk while cooking gives this recipe some creaminess without being too heavy or congestive for Kapha.

3 cups water

1 cup Tridoshic Almond Milk (page 57)

⅔ cup quinoa

4 egg whites (optional)

2 teaspoons ground cinnamon, plus for serving

½ teaspoon ground ginger

¼ teaspoon cardamom powder

½ teaspoon vanilla extract

1 teaspoon ghee

6 tablespoons Morning Energy Mix (page 180), divided

2 to 4 teaspoons maple syrup

Splash almond milk, for serving

1. In a medium saucepan, heat the water and almond milk to just below a boil.

2. While the water and milk are heating, put the quinoa into a spice grinder or blender and grind it into a fine powder.

3. Once the water and almond milk are just about to boil, reduce the heat to low. Slowly sprinkle in the quinoa while stirring continuously. Stir out any lumps that form. If a hand blender is available, simply pour the quinoa into the pan all at once and blend out any lumps that form.

4. Cook, mostly covered, on low for 8 minutes, stirring every 2 minutes. If the porridge becomes too thick, add more water by the tablespoon.

5. In a small bowl, whisk 4 egg whites (if using). Add the egg whites to the quinoa and stir well for 1 minute.

6. Turn off the heat, but leave the pan on the warm burner. Add the cinnamon, ginger, cardamom, vanilla, ghee, and 4 tablespoons of the Morning Energy Mix. Stir well, cover, and let sit for 2 minutes.

7. Serve into bowls. Top each bowl with 1 to 2 teaspoons of maple syrup, a splash of almond milk, 1 tablespoon of Morning Energy Mix, and a sprinkle of cinnamon.

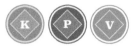

# Quinoa Breakfast Smoothie

**GOOD FOR:** Energy, Digestion, Constipation, Heart Health, Blood Sugar Balance, Pregnancy, Postpartum, Lactation

**MAKES 2 CUPS / PREP TIME: 15 MINUTES**

Here is a deliciously healing smoothie for all body types to enjoy. Made using precooked quinoa, it can be enjoyed warm during the cooler months, and at room temperature when it's hot. It is grounding, yet not too heavy, leaving you energized and ready to start your day.

2 medjool dates, pitted and soaked (use 1 date for Kapha)

1 cup Tridoshic Almond Milk (page 57)

1 cup cooked quinoa

¼ cup plain yogurt (use goat milk or almond milk yogurt for Kapha)

¼ teaspoon ground ginger

½ teaspoon ground cinnamon, plus for serving

⅛ teaspoon cardamom powder

2 tablespoons Morning Energy Mix (page 180)

1 teaspoon cacao powder (optional; omit for Vata)

1 teaspoon honey (optional; use maple syrup for Pitta)

½ teaspoon vanilla extract

**1.** Put the dates, almond milk, quinoa, yogurt, ginger, cinnamon, cardamom, Morning Energy Mix, cacao, honey, and vanilla into a blender.

**2.** Blend on high for 2 to 3 minutes, or until a completely smooth texture has been reached.

**3.** Place the smoothie into a glass or mug, and sprinkle with a dash of cinnamon.

**4.** Sit, sip, energize, and enjoy!

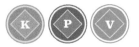

# Golden Energy
# Buckwheat Breakfast

**GOOD FOR:** Digestion, Constipation, Colon Health, Heart Health, High Cholesterol, High Blood Pressure, Weight Loss, Pregnancy, Postpartum

**SERVES 2 / PREP TIME: 5 MINUTES / COOK TIME: 20 MINUTES**

Kapha types do well with buckwheat due to its light quality. It's also healing for Pitta due to its cooling property, and balancing for Vata due to its soft, easy-to-digest nature. This porridge boosts overall heart health.

2 cups water

1 cup raw buckwheat groats

Pinch salt

1 cup Tridoshic Almond Milk (page 57)

½ teaspoon turmeric powder

1 teaspoon ground cinnamon, plus for serving

1 teaspoon ashwagandha (optional)

½ teaspoon ground ginger

¼ teaspoon cardamom powder

30 raisins

2 teaspoons shredded coconut (omit or use 1 teaspoon for Kapha)

1 teaspoon ghee

Splash Tridoshic Almond Milk

2 to 4 teaspoons honey (use maple syrup for Pitta)

2 tablespoons Morning Energy Mix (page 180), divided

1. In a small saucepan, bring the water to a boil. Reduce the heat to low and stir in the buckwheat groats and a pinch of salt.

2. Cook, mostly covered, for 15 minutes. Stir every 5 minutes.

3. Stir in the almond milk, turmeric, cinnamon, ashwagandha (if using), ginger, cardamom, raisins, coconut, and ghee. Stirring frequently, cook, covered, for an additional 2 to 3 minutes, or until the buckwheat obtains the desired softness.

4. Serve into bowls. Top each bowl with almond milk, 1 to 2 teaspoons of honey, 1 tablespoon of Morning Energy Mix, and a dash of cinnamon.

# Kapha-Reducing Millet Porridge

**GOOD FOR:** Digestion, Colon Health, Heart Health, Liver Health, Kidney Health, Congestion, High Cholesterol, High Blood Pressure, Weight Loss, Pregnancy, Postpartum

**SERVES 2 / PREP TIME: 5 MINUTES / COOK TIME: 25 MINUTES**

Similar to quinoa in shape and size, millet has a drier and crunchier texture. This makes it great for Kaphas. This porridge makes for an energizing breakfast when you're experiencing congestion, slow metabolism, sluggish digestion, or general lethargy.

2 cups water

2 cups Tridoshic Almond Milk (page 57), divided

⅔ cup millet

2 cinnamon sticks

15 to 20 raisins

1 tablespoon slivered almonds

1 teaspoon ground cinnamon, plus for serving

½ teaspoon ground ginger

⅛ teaspoon cardamom powder

4 tablespoons Morning Energy Mix (page 180), divided

4 teaspoons honey, divided

1. In a medium saucepan, bring the water and 1 cup of almond milk to a boil.

2. Once they're boiling, reduce the heat to medium-low and add the millet and cinnamon sticks. Cook, mostly covered, for 20 to 22 minutes, stirring every 5 minutes.

3. Turn off the heat, but let the pan sit on the hot burner. Add the remaining 1 cup of almond milk along with the raisins, almonds, cinnamon, ginger, cardamom, and 2 tablespoons of Morning Energy Mix.

4. Cover the pan and let the porridge sit for 5 minutes.

5. Serve into bowls. Once the porridge has cooled slightly, add 1 to 2 teaspoons of honey per bowl.

6. Top each bowl with a dash of cinnamon and 1 tablespoon of the remaining Morning Energy Mix.

7. Eat with awareness and gratitude as you begin your beautiful day.

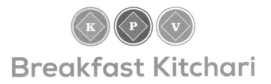

# Breakfast Kitchari

**GOOD FOR:** Digestion, Detox, Constipation, Colon Health, Heart Health, High Cholesterol, High Blood Pressure, Weight Loss, Pregnancy, Postpartum

**SERVES 2 / PREP TIME: 5 MINUTES / COOK TIME: 25 MINUTES**

Kitchari is a very versatile dish and just by switching up a few ingredients, it can be made into a sweet, nourishing breakfast. This recipe can help you with digestive imbalance, detoxification, post-cleansing, post-illness, general weakness, and weight loss.

3 cups water

⅔ cup mung dal

1 cinnamon stick

Large pinch salt

½ cup basmati rice

½ cup grated carrots

½ teaspoon turmeric powder

1 teaspoon ground cinnamon

⅛ teaspoon cardamom powder

¼ teaspoon ground ginger

4 dates, pitted and chopped (use 2 for Kapha)

2 tablespoons cashew pieces

1 tablespoon shredded coconut (omit for Kapha), plus for serving

2 teaspoons ghee

2 to 4 teaspoons honey (maple syrup for Pitta)

1. In a medium saucepan, bring the water to a boil. Reduce the heat to medium-low. Stir in the mung dal, cinnamon stick, and salt.

2. Cook, mostly covered, for 10 minutes, stirring at the halfway point.

3. Add the basmati rice and grated carrots. Stir well and replace the cover, cooking for 15 minutes. Stir every 5 minutes.

4. Turn the heat off but leave the pan on the hot burner. Add the turmeric, cinnamon, cardamom, ginger, dates, cashews, coconut, and ghee. Cover the pan completely and let sit for 5 minutes.

5. Serve into bowls. Once the kitchari has cooled slightly, add 1 to 2 teaspoons of honey per bowl and sprinkle with cinnamon and coconut.

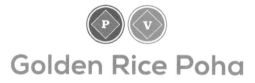

# Golden Rice Poha

**GOOD FOR:** Digestion, Energy, Immunity, Circulation, Heart Health, High Cholesterol, Weight Loss, Pregnancy, Postpartum

**SERVES 3 TO 4 / PREP TIME: 5 MINUTES / COOK TIME: 20 MINUTES**

Poha is flattened basmati rice sautéed with potato, onion, and spices to make a deliciously savory Indian breakfast. This particular Poha recipe replaces the flattened rice with golden rice, creating a fusion of sweet and savory. If you are looking to make this meal Kapha-balancing, simply replace the basmati rice with an equal amount of quinoa and enjoy!

### For the rice

2 cups water

Large pinch salt

⅛ teaspoon freshly ground black pepper

1 to 2 cinnamon sticks

¼ teaspoon cardamom powder

¼ teaspoon turmeric powder

4 saffron threads

2 teaspoons ghee, divided

1 cup basmati rice

### For the sauté

1 teaspoon of ghee

½ cup sweet onion, minced

½ teaspoon cumin seeds, whole

½ teaspoon brown mustard seeds, whole (omit for Pitta)

⅛ teaspoon freshly ground black pepper

1 teaspoon serrano pepper, finely minced (optional; omit for Pitta)

2 tablespoons cashew pieces

⅛ teaspoon turmeric powder

1 teaspoon finely minced fresh ginger

1 cup unpeeled potato, chopped

¼ cup water

2 tablespoons minced cilantro leaf

2 tablespoons shredded coconut

Juice of ½ lime

Large pinch of salt

**To make the rice**

1. In a medium saucepan, bring the water, salt, pepper, cinnamon sticks, cardamom, turmeric, saffron, and 1 teaspoon of ghee to a boil. Reduce the heat to medium-low.

2. Add the basmati rice and cook, mostly covered, for 10 to 12 minutes.

3. Turn the heat off, but leave the pan on the hot burner. Stir in the remaining 1 teaspoon of ghee and cover for 5 minutes.

**To make the sauté**

1. In a large sauté pan or skillet, heat the ghee over medium heat. Then add the onion, cumin, brown mustard seeds, and black pepper. Sauté for 2 minutes, stirring frequently.

2. Add the serrano pepper (if using), cashews, turmeric, and ginger. Stir well and sauté for 1 minute.

3. Add the potato and water and sauté for 5 to 7 minutes, stirring frequently. For a softer texture, cover the pan after adding the water (recommended for Vata).

4. Once the potatoes are fork-tender, turn off the heat, but leave the pan on the hot burner. Add the golden rice and stir well.

5. Add the cilantro, coconut, and lime juice. Sprinkle with salt and blend well. Enjoy warm.

# Sweet Potato Scramble Chapati Wrap

**GOOD FOR:** Energy, Digestion, Skin Health, Eye Health, Heart Health, Pregnancy, Postpartum

**SERVES 2 / PREP TIME: 10 MINUTES / COOK TIME: 15 TO 20 MINUTES**

This lovely scramble lets you switch up your breakfast routine with a bit of heartiness—without heaviness. It provides you with energy and strength, and leaves you feeling satiated. Feel free to replace the chapati with a whole-grain tortilla.

3 teaspoons ghee, divided

½ teaspoon cumin seeds, whole

¼ teaspoon brown mustard seeds, whole (omit for Pitta)

⅛ teaspoon freshly ground black pepper

1 small sweet potato, chopped (¼-inch cubes)

6 kale leaves, stemmed and chopped (use 3 cups chopped spinach for Vata)

¼ cup water

3 whole eggs

3 egg whites

Large pinch salt

2 pieces Essential Chapati (page 93) (or whole-grain tortilla)

1. In a large sauté pan or skillet, heat 2 teaspoons of ghee over medium heat. Add the cumin seeds, brown mustard seeds, and black pepper. Sauté for 2 minutes, stirring frequently.

2. Add the sweet potato and stir well. Sauté for 2 minutes, stirring frequently.

3. Add the kale and water. Stir well. Continue to cook for 5 to 7 minutes, stirring every 1 to 2 minutes.

4. While the veggies are cooking, whisk the eggs and egg whites together in a small bowl.

5. Once you have reached a desirable softness for the veggies, cover the pan and set it aside.

6. In a medium sauté pan or skillet, heat the remaining 1 teaspoon of ghee over medium heat. Pour in the eggs and stir well. Cook for 2 to 3 minutes or until fully cooked, stirring frequently.

7. Add the eggs to the sweet potato and kale blend. Add salt and stir well.

8. Warm a precooked chapati (or tortilla) in a sauté pan for several seconds per side.

9. Place the chapati onto a plate, and pour the scramble into the center. Roll up the sides to form a wrap or a burrito.

10. Sit, breathe, and enjoy in good company.

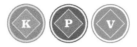

# Springtime Breakfast Scramble

**GOOD FOR:** Energy, Digestion, Constipation, Heart Health, Weight Loss, Pregnancy, Postpartum

**SERVES 4 / PREP TIME: 15 MINUTES / COOK TIME: 15 MINUTES**

This colorful scramble gives you a light and healthy breakfast option for the spring and summer months. Using a wide variety of seasonal vegetables, this delicious dish makes it easy to sneak some extra nutrients into your breakfast.

**For the quinoa**

2 cups water

1 cup quinoa

¼ teaspoon turmeric powder

⅛ teaspoon salt

2 teaspoons ghee

**For the scramble**

4 teaspoons ghee, divided

½ teaspoon whole cumin seeds

¼ teaspoon brown mustard seeds whole (omit for Pitta)

⅛ teaspoon freshly ground black pepper

½ teaspoon turmeric powder

¼ teaspoon salt

1 zucchini, chopped

1 yellow squash, chopped

½ red pepper, chopped

6 asparagus spears, chopped

2 cups chopped kale, loosely packed

2 whole eggs

6 egg whites

**To make the quinoa**

1. In a small saucepan, bring the water to a boil.

2. Reduce the heat to low and add the quinoa, turmeric, salt, and ghee.

3. Cook, mostly covered, on low for 15 minutes.

4. Cover and set aside until the sauté is complete.

**To make the scramble**

1. Heat 2 teaspoons of ghee in a large sauté pan or skillet over medium heat. Add the cumin seeds, brown mustard seeds, and black pepper. Sauté for 2 minutes, stirring frequently. Add the turmeric and salt and sauté for 30 seconds.

2. Add the zucchini, yellow squash, red pepper, asparagus, and kale. Stir well.

3. Sauté, uncovered, over medium heat for 5 minutes. Stir frequently.

4. Cover and cook for 2 minutes or until the veggies are cooked to your preference. If you prefer vegetables more steamed, add 1 to 2 tablespoons of water before covering (recommended for Vata types).

5. Once the veggies are cooked, set them aside in a bowl.

6. Whisk the whole eggs and egg whites in a separate bowl.

7. In the large sauté pan, heat the remaining 2 teaspoons of ghee over medium heat.

8. Pour in the eggs. Cook while stirring frequently for about 2 minutes or until the eggs are fully cooked. They should not be dry or runny.

9. Turn off the heat, but keep the pan on the hot burner. Add the sautéed veggies and the cooked quinoa and blend evenly.

10. Serve into bowls. Add any additional salt, pepper, and ghee as desired.

11. Eat, share, and enjoy!

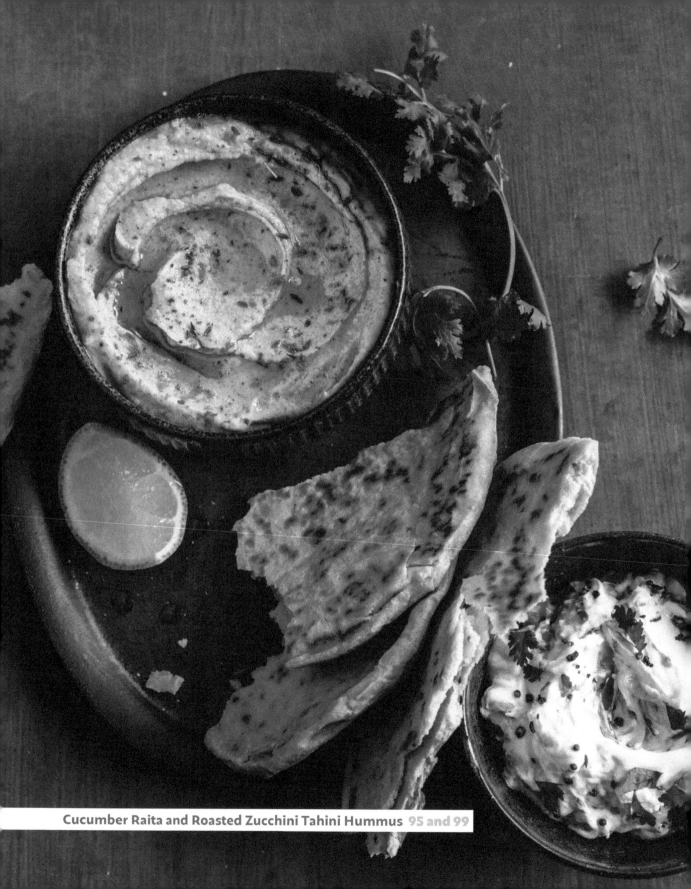

**Cucumber Raita and Roasted Zucchini Tahini Hummus  95 and 99**

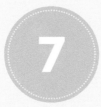

# SIDES, SNACKS, AND DIPS

# Everyday Basmati Rice

**GOOD FOR:** Digestion, Energy, Constipation, Pregnancy, Postpartum, Lactation

**SERVES 5 TO 6 / COOK TIME: 15 TO 20 MINUTES**

Basmati rice is essential when it comes to Ayurvedic cooking: It's cooling for Pitta and soothing for Vata, making it a great dietary staple. Due to its sticky nature, however, it can be a bit heavy for many Kapha types. Kapha types should go for lighter whole grains such as quinoa, millet, or buckwheat.

2 cups water

1 cup Indian basmati rice (see Ingredient Tip)

2 teaspoons ghee, divided

⅛ teaspoon freshly ground black pepper

Pinch salt

1. In a medium saucepan, bring the water to a boil.

2. Reduce the heat to low and stir in the basmati rice, 1 teaspoon of ghee, the black pepper, and the salt. Cook, mostly covered, for 12 minutes, covering completely with the lid around 6 minutes.

3. Turn off the heat, but leave the pan on the hot burner. Add the remaining 1 teaspoon of ghee and stir well. Cover the pan and let sit for 5 minutes.

4. Stir the rice and serve as a light snack, a side dish, or as part of your main meal.

**INGREDIENT TIP:**

*It is best to get aged (ideally 5 years or more) Indian grown basmati rice, which can be found in Indian markets, international markets, or online.*

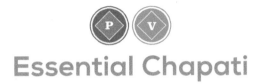

# Essential Chapati

**MAKES 8 / PREP TIME: 20 MINUTES / COOK TIME: 10 MINUTES**

Chapati is an Indian flatbread and considered a staple for savory meals. This Essential Chapati recipe wonderfully complements just about any lunch or dinner recipe in this book. This recipe uses 100 percent whole wheat flour, providing more flavor and vital nutrients. Whole wheat is cooling, strengthening, and energizing, making it an ideal option for balancing Vata and Pitta, although Kaphas can also enjoy it in moderation.

¾ teaspoon salt

2½ cups 100 percent whole wheat flour

¾ cup warm water, divided

1 tablespoon ghee

1. In a medium mixing bowl, blend the salt and flour evenly.

2. Add the water and the ghee and mix evenly. You want a moist dough that is not sticky, nor crumbly. If the dough sticks to your hands, add more flour. If the dough is not able to hold a ball form without cracking, add water carefully by the tablespoon.

3. Once you find the perfect texture, knead the dough for 5 minutes.

4. Cut the dough into 8 even portions. This will give you about 8-inch-round chapatis. If you prefer smaller chapatis, increase the number of portions.

5. Roll each section into a ball.

6. Lightly flour your countertop. Using a rolling pin, roll out one of the balls.

continued ▸

7. The final chapati dough should be very thin, similar to the thickness of a tortilla. The shape doesn't need to be a perfect circle.

8. While rolling, begin to heat an ungreased large griddle or sauté pan over medium-high heat.

9. Put one rolled-out chapati completely flat onto the heated pan.

10. Cook the first side for 15 to 30 seconds, or until bubbles start to form in the dough. Flip over and cook for another 15 to 30 seconds. Then flip one last time and cook for a final 15 to 20 seconds. If the cooked chapati is hard or rubbery, you are likely cooking it too long. They should be soft and flexible.

11. Repeat this process with the remaining uncooked chapatis.

12. Chapati is best when eaten immediately to enjoy the softest texture and freshest flavor. However, they will keep for up to 2 to 3 hours when covered tightly with foil and stored in an unheated oven.

### STORAGE TIP:

*Cooked chapatis can be stored in the freezer for up to 3 months. Wrap each one individually in plastic wrap and then again in foil. Before reheating, place the frozen chapati in the refrigerator for several hours to thaw. Then heat the chapatis in a sauté pan over medium-high heat for 10 seconds per side or until warm. Serve immediately.*

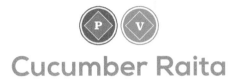

# Cucumber Raita

**MAKES 2 CUPS / PREP TIME: 20 MINUTES / COOK TIME: 5 MINUTES**

Cucumber raita is typically eaten as a side to dal, curries, rice dishes, vegetables, and flatbreads. This creamy condiment is cooling, hydrating, nutrient-rich, and filled with gut-healing probiotics. It can help you improve your digestion and soothe inflammation, especially in the GI tract.

1 large cucumber, seeded and grated (skin on)

1 teaspoon ghee

½ teaspoon cumin powder

¼ teaspoon brown mustard seeds, whole (omit for Pitta)

⅛ teaspoon freshly ground black pepper

1 teaspoon finely minced fresh ginger

1 teaspoon finely minced serrano pepper (omit for Pitta)

1½ cups plain yogurt

2 tablespoons minced cilantro, packed

¼ teaspoon salt

1. Take a paper towel and squeeze the grated cucumber to remove any excess water.

2. In a small sauté pan or skillet, heat the ghee over medium heat. Add the cumin, brown mustard seeds, and black pepper and sauté for 2 minutes. Add the ginger and serrano pepper and sauté for 1 minute more.

3. In a medium mixing bowl, combine the yogurt, cucumber, sautéed spice mixture, cilantro, and salt. Mix the ingredients together evenly.

4. Serve a small amount on the side of any meal as a cooling condiment or creamy salad.

5. Store in an airtight container in the refrigerator for up to 4 days.

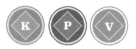

# Traditional Digestion Lassi

**GOOD FOR:** Digestion, Energy, Bone Health, Pregnancy, Postpartum, Lactation

**MAKES 2½ CUPS / PREP TIME: 10 MINUTES**

The combination of healing spices and probiotics in this tridoshic lassi is perfect for boosting digestion and promoting healthy gut flora. Drink a half cup after a meal or between meals, twice a day on a consistent basis. Whenever possible, use fresh, homemade yogurt.

½ cup plain yogurt (use goat yogurt or non-dairy yogurt for Kapha)

2 cups water

½ teaspoon cumin powder

¼ teaspoon ground ginger

¼ teaspoon fennel powder

⅛ teaspoon freshly ground black pepper

2 teaspoons finely minced cilantro leaf

1. Put the yogurt and water into a large jar with a lid.

2. Add the cumin, ginger, fennel, pepper, and cilantro. If time permits, the spices can be dry roasted.

3. Mix all the ingredients together using a hand blender or spoon, or simply shake the closed jar. Blend evenly.

4. Store in an airtight jar in the refrigerator for up to 5 days. Shake well before serving.

# Golden Spiced Sweet Lassi

**GOOD FOR:** Digestion, Energy, Skin Health, Liver Health, Bone Health, Anemia, Inflammation, Pregnancy, Postpartum, Lactation

**MAKES 1½ CUPS / PREP TIME: 10 MINUTES**

This lassi gets its sweetness from coconut water and honey. Turmeric and ginger further enhance the flavor and healing properties. Enjoy it directly after a meal or as a healthy snack between meals to reduce symptoms such as gas, bloating, and indigestion.

½ cup plain yogurt (use goat yogurt or non-dairy yogurt for Kapha)

1 cup coconut water

⅛ teaspoon turmeric powder

¼ teaspoon ground ginger

Large pinch cardamom powder

4 saffron threads

¼ teaspoon vanilla extract

1 teaspoon honey (use maple syrup for Pitta)

**1.** Combine the yogurt, coconut water, turmeric, ginger, cardamom, saffron, vanilla, and honey in a large jar, and blend evenly with a spoon or hand blender.

**2.** If time permits, let this mixture sit for 10 minutes to allow the spices to steep. Stir well before serving.

**3.** Drink ½ cup of the lassi directly after a meal or between meals.

**4.** Store in an airtight jar in the refrigerator for up to 5 days.

# Coconut Curry Hummus

**GOOD FOR:** Energy, Weight Loss, High Cholesterol, High Blood Pressure, Heart Health, Colon Health, Pregnancy, Postpartum, Lactation

**MAKES 2 CUPS / PREP TIME: 15 MINUTES**

If you need a healthy, tasty, savory snack for the spring and summer seasons, this is it! With its high protein and fiber content, hummus is beneficial for weight loss, lowering cholesterol levels, controlling your appetite, and promoting healthy digestion and elimination.

¼ cup coconut water

1 tablespoon olive oil

Juice of 1 lime

¼ cup chopped cilantro

½ teaspoon cumin powder

½ teaspoon turmeric powder

⅛ teaspoon cayenne pepper (optional; omit for Pitta)

¼ teaspoon salt

2 tablespoons tahini

1 (15-ounce) can chickpeas (1½ cups cooked)

1. Put the coconut water, olive oil, and lime juice in a blender.

2. Add the cilantro, cumin, turmeric, cayenne pepper (if using), salt, tahini, and chickpeas.

3. Blend on high for 2 to 3 minutes or until the hummus is completely smooth and creamy. If needed, add a splash of coconut water.

4. Enjoy this as a veggie dip, a spread, or alone. Hummus makes a healthy snack option for Pitta and Kapha types during warmer seasons.

5. Store in an airtight container in the refrigerator for up to 6 days.

**PAIRING TIP:**

*This hummus recipe will be a great complement to Summertime Salad (page 122), Simply Delicious Lettuce Wrap (page 123), and Essential Chapati (page 93).*

# Roasted Zucchini Tahini Hummus

**GOOD FOR:** Weight Loss, Appetite Control, High Cholesterol, Blood Sugar Balance, Digestion Health, Colon Health, Energy, Anemia, Circulation

**MAKES 3 CUPS / PREP TIME: 15 MINUTES / COOK TIME: 15 MINUTES**

Hummus helps you control your appetite and keep your blood sugar levels stable. This recipe uses roasted zucchini, yellow squash, and tahini for optimal flavor, texture, and health benefits.

1 medium zucchini, chopped

1 medium yellow squash, chopped

2 tablespoons olive oil, divided

3 tablespoons Golden Tahini Sauce (page 184) (substitute with plain tahini)

3 tablespoons fresh lemon juice

¾ teaspoon cumin seeds

¼ teaspoon turmeric powder

⅛ teaspoon freshly ground black pepper

¾ teaspoon salt

⅛ teaspoon cayenne pepper (optional; omit for Pitta)

1 (15-ounce) can chickpeas (1½ cups cooked)

1. Preheat the oven to 425°F.

2. Put the zucchini and squash in a glass baking dish. Pour 1 tablespoon olive oil over the veggies and stir until evenly coated.

3. Roast for 10 to 12 minutes, stirring at the halfway point.

4. After 10 minutes, check on the squash mixture. The pieces should be a bit toasted, juicy, and slightly soft all the way through.

5. Put the veggies in a blender. In this order, add the remaining 1 tablespoon of olive oil, the tahini sauce, lemon juice, cumin seeds, turmeric, black pepper, salt, cayenne pepper (if using), and chickpeas.

6. Blend on high for 2 to 3 minutes or until everything is completely smooth. Taste the hummus and add extra salt, lemon juice, or spices as needed.

7. Your hummus will be warm. If preferred, cool it in the refrigerator for 1 to 2 hours before enjoying.

# Creamy Tahini Broth

**GOOD FOR:** Energy, Immunity, Digestion, Constipation, Bone Health, Arthritis, Inflammation, Skin Health, Pregnancy, Postpartum, Lactation

**MAKES 6 CUPS / COOK TIME: 10 MINUTES**

This Creamy Tahini Broth is an energizing and strengthening tonic that is great for Vata imbalance, low immunity, illness, constipation, depletion, malabsorption, post-cleansing, pregnancy, and postpartum. This warming recipe is perfect for maintaining optimal health throughout the cooler seasons.

6 cups bone broth, chicken broth, or veggie broth (unsalted)

½ cup tahini

1½ tablespoons Vata Masala (page 178)

Juice of ½ lemon

Small pinch cayenne pepper (optional)

Pinch freshly ground black pepper

⅛ teaspoon salt

Chopped scallions (green parts), for garnish

1. In a large saucepan, heat the broth to just below a boil.

2. Reduce the heat to low and add the tahini, Vata Masala, lemon juice, cayenne pepper (if using), black pepper, and salt. Blend well using a hand blender, or allow to cool slightly and transfer to a blender to process.

3. Serve into small bowls and top with scallions.

4. Enjoy this broth as a nourishing snack or pair it with some rice, quinoa, or steamed veggies to make a meal. Store any extra in the refrigerator for up to 6 days.

# Cooling Coconut and Kale Sauté

**GOOD FOR:** Digestion, Constipation, Detox, Excessive Heat, Inflammation, Liver Health, Skin Health, Heart Health, Cancer Prevention

**SERVES 4 TO 6 / PREP TIME: 10 MINUTES / COOK TIME: 10 MINUTES**

With its bitter taste and cooling, anti-inflammatory properties, kale is a great choice for Pitta types and Pitta conditions like eczema, psoriasis, acne, and excessive heat. Kale's light, dry, and rough qualities also make this recipe ideal for Kaphas. This sauté is helpful for weight loss, congestion, high cholesterol, slow metabolism, heaviness, and fatigue.

1 tablespoon coconut oil

½ teaspoon cumin seeds, whole

1 tablespoon almond slivers

1 teaspoon Pitta Masala (page 177) (replace with ¼ teaspoon turmeric powder)

1 tablespoon finely minced fresh ginger

1 bunch kale, stems removed, roughly chopped

¼ cup water

2 tablespoons shredded coconut

Juice of ½ lime

⅛ teaspoon salt

1. In a large sauté pan or skillet, heat the coconut oil over medium heat. Add the cumin seeds and slivered almonds. Sauté for 2 minutes, stirring frequently. Add the Pitta Masala and ginger, and sauté for another 30 seconds.

2. Add the kale and the water. Cook for 4 to 5 minutes, stirring continuously.

3. Add the shredded coconut, and cook for an additional 30 seconds, stirring continuously.

4. Turn off the heat, but keep the pan on the hot burner. Add the lime juice and salt, and blend evenly.

5. Serve this dish as a light dinner, a healthy snack, or as a side dish.

**PAIRING TIP:**

*This cooling kale dish pairs well with the Pressure Cooker Mung Dal (page 110).*

# Kapha-Reducing Kale Chips

**GOOD FOR:** Digestion, Constipation, Weight Loss, Detox, Liver Health, Skin Health, Heart Health, Cancer Prevention

**SERVES 2 / PREP TIME: 15 MINUTES / COOK TIME: 15 MINUTES**

Kale chips make an excellent snack for Kaphas during the spring and summer. With just the right amount of healthy oil, digestive spices, and sunflower seed topping, these cooling, crispy treats help with sluggish digestion, weight loss, detoxification, congestion, and general feelings of heaviness.

1 bunch kale

2 tablespoons sunflower seeds, finely ground

2 teaspoons Tridoshic Masala (page 179)

2 tablespoons sunflower oil

Juice of ½ lime

Pinch of cayenne pepper (optional; omit for Pitta)

Pink Himalayan salt

1. Preheat the oven to 300°F.
2. Wash the kale and dry each leaf thoroughly.
3. Remove the stems from the kale, and pull apart each leaf into 2-inch pieces. Place them in a large mixing bowl.
4. In a spice grinder or blender, grind the sunflower seeds to a fine powder.
5. In a small bowl, combine the ground sunflower seeds, Tridoshic Masala, sunflower oil, lime juice, and cayenne pepper (if using). Stir well to make a thin paste.
6. Drizzle the sunflower oil mixture onto the kale pieces, and rub each leaf to cover evenly. There should be no dry spots on any of the kale pieces.

7. Place the coated kale pieces onto two cookie sheets. Flatten and separate each piece for the crispiest results. Sprinkle lightly with salt.

8. Bake for 7 minutes. After 7 minutes, rotate the cookie sheets and cook for 6 more minutes.

9. Check on the chips. If they are not mildly crispy, keep them in the oven and check on them every minute until they have reached the desired crispiness. (The chips crisp a bit more after sitting out, so taking them out a bit less crispy is much better than having them overly crispy—or burnt!) Finished chips should be crunchy with a touch of moisture. They should retain the bright green color with no burnt taste.

10. Once done, let the kale chips sit for 5 minutes before transferring them onto a plate.

11. Eat, share, and indulge in good company!

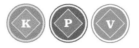

# Ojas-Increasing Energy Balls

**GOOD FOR:** Energy, Immunity, Libido, Skin Health, Hair Health, Heart Health, Brain Health, Pregnancy, Postpartum, Lactation

**MAKES 18 BALLS / PREP TIME: 20 MINUTES (PLUS TIME IN THE FREEZER)**

This Ayurvedic twist on everyday energy balls will leave your sweet tooth satiated and your body energized. Delicious spices increase digestion and metabolism, reduce inflammation, and stimulate the mind. The ashwagandha root enhances energy and immunity.

¾ cup almonds

¼ cup pumpkin seeds

¼ cup sunflower seeds

2 tablespoons cacao powder (omit for Vata)

⅓ cup plus 2 tablespoons shredded coconut, divided

2 tablespoons ashwagandha root powder (optional, but recommended)

1 teaspoon ground cinnamon

1 teaspoon ground ginger

½ teaspoon turmeric powder

¼ teaspoon cardamom powder

⅛ teaspoon salt

¼ cup honey (use maple syrup for Pitta)

2 tablespoons almond butter

2 tablespoons ghee (use 1 tablespoon for Kapha)

1. Grind up the almonds, pumpkin seeds, and sunflower seeds in a blender or food processor until they become a fine powder.

2. In a large mixing bowl, combine the ground nut powder, cacao, 2 tablespoons of coconut, ashwagandha (if using), cinnamon, ginger, turmeric, cardamom, and salt. Blend evenly.

3. Add the honey, almond butter, and ghee. Using clean hands, mix everything together until well blended.

4. Take a small amount of the batter, and begin to roll it in the palms of your hands. Put the completed ball onto a plate, and continue to roll the batter until it is used up.

5. Place the remaining ⅓ cup of shredded coconut in a small bowl.

6. Roll each ball in the coconut until it is fully coated. Repeat this step until all the balls have been coated.

7. Once you are done, place the balls in the freezer for 1 to 2 hours to get them nice and solid before serving.

8. Store in an airtight container in the freezer for up to 3 months.

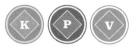

# Spiced Apples and Ghee

**GOOD FOR:** Diarrhea, Constipation, Digestion, Energy, Heart Health, Weight Loss, Pregnancy, Postpartum

**SERVES 2 / PREP TIME: 5 MINUTES / COOK TIME: 10 MINUTES**

Apples are essential for keeping your digestion strong and your elimination regular. They are useful for alleviating constipation, yet equally as effective for treating diarrhea and loose stools. This tridoshic recipe can be enjoyed anytime of year, although it is best during fall and winter months when apples are the most fresh.

2 tablespoons ghee

2 apples, chopped into small cubes

1 tablespoon water

½ teaspoon ground cinnamon

¼ teaspoon ground ginger

⅛ teaspoon cardamom powder

⅛ teaspoon vanilla extract

1. In a large sauté pan or skillet, heat the ghee over medium-low heat.

2. Add the apples and water. Sauté the apples, uncovered, for 5 minutes, stirring frequently.

3. Sprinkle in the cinnamon, ginger, and cardamom. Stir well, making sure the apples become evenly coated. Cook for 1 minute.

4. Remove the pan from the heat and add the vanilla. Stir evenly.

5. Sit, share, and enjoy this soothing snack for the soul.

6. Store any extra in an airtight container in the refrigerator for up to 5 days.

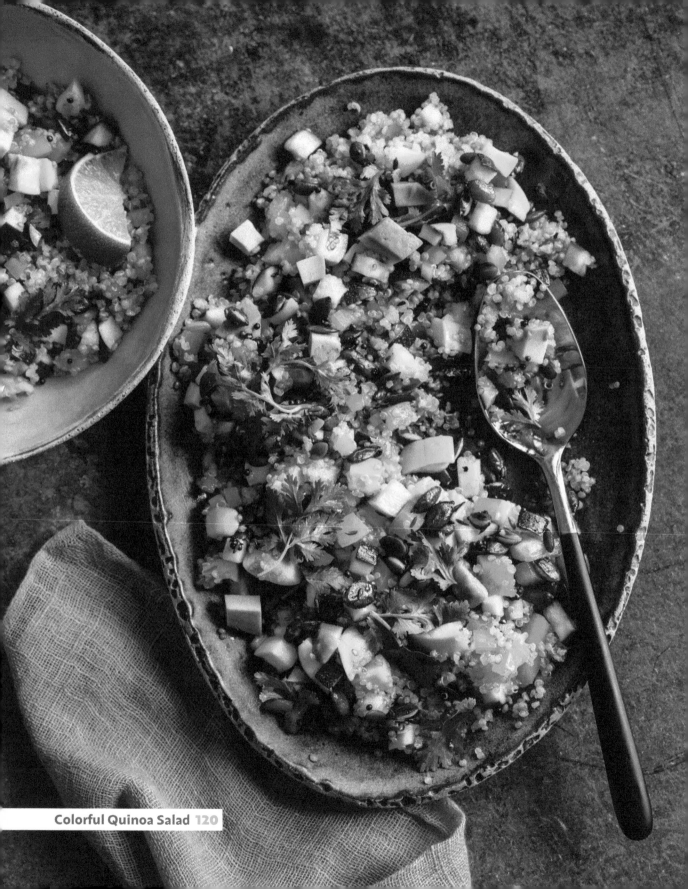

Colorful Quinoa Salad 120

# LUNCHES

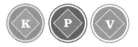

# Perfect Pressure Cooker Mung Dal

**GOOD FOR:** Digestion, Detox, Constipation, Energy, Weight Loss, Colon Health, Heart Health, Immunity, Mental Balance, Pregnancy, Postpartum

**SERVES 2 TO 4 / PREP TIME: 5 MINUTES / COOK TIME: 15 MINUTES**

A diet rich in mung dal promotes a strong body, calm mind, and healthy digestion. One of the most satvic (balanced), life-promoting foods, mung dal can be eaten all year round. It pairs amazingly well with Cooling Coconut and Kale Sauté (page 101), Sautéed Kale and Golden Tahini Sauce (page 119), and Curried Cauliflower, Potato, and Kale Subji (page 117).

1 cup mung dal

1 tablespoon ghee

¼ cup minced onion

½ teaspoon cumin seeds, whole

½ teaspoon brown mustard seeds, whole (omit for Pitta)

¼ teaspoon freshly ground black pepper

¼ teaspoon fennel seeds, whole

2 tablespoons finely minced fresh ginger

2 tablespoons shredded coconut (omit for Kapha)

½ teaspoon Tridoshic Masala (page 179) or turmeric powder

⅛ teaspoon cayenne pepper (optional; omit for Pitta)

3½ cups water

Chopped cilantro leaf, for garnish

Chopped scallions (green parts), for garnish

1. Rinse the mung dal in warm water. Strain and set aside.

2. In an open stovetop pressure cooker, heat the ghee over medium heat.

3. Add the onion, cumin seeds, brown mustard seeds, black pepper, and fennel seeds. Sauté over medium-low heat for 2 minutes, stirring frequently.

4. Add the ginger, coconut, Tridoshic Masala (or turmeric), and the cayenne pepper (if using). Continue to sauté for 1 minute, stirring constantly.

5. Add the water and mung dal, stir well, and cover the pressure cooker.

6. Cook on high for 5 to 6 minutes, or until the pressure cooker begins to whistle.

7. Reduce the heat to low and cook for 5 minutes.

8. Turn the heat off, but leave the pressure cooker on the hot burner. Let sit covered for 10 minutes to allow most of the pressure to release naturally.

9. Carefully open the pressure cooker and stir well. Garnish with cilantro and scallions, and serve.

# Quick and Easy Sambar

**GOOD FOR:** Digestion, Detox, Weight Loss, Anemia, Liver Health, Skin Health, Immunity, Pregnancy, Postpartum

**SERVES 4 TO 6 / PREP TIME: 5 MINUTES / COOK TIME: 25 MINUTES**

Sambar is a traditional South Indian vegetable and dal soup. It is soupier than a typical dal and thicker than a typical soup. This recipe uses the Tridoshic Masala instead of sambar powder, mung dal instead of tur dal, and tamarind paste instead of fresh tamarind to keep the prep easy.

**For the dal**

2 cups water

¾ cup mung dal

1 tablespoon coconut oil

**For the sambar**

2 tablespoons coconut oil

¼ cup minced onion

½ teaspoon cumin seeds, whole

½ teaspoon brown mustard seeds, whole

¼ teaspoon freshly ground black pepper

½ teaspoon salt, divided

¼ teaspoon turmeric powder

⅛ teaspoon cayenne pepper (optional)

½ teaspoon finely minced serrano pepper

2 tablespoons finely minced fresh ginger

5 curry leaves or 2 bay leaves

3⅓ cups water, divided

⅓ cup chopped beets

½ cup chopped yellow squash

¼ cup thinly sliced carrots

1 tablespoon tamarind paste

1½ cups coarsely packed chopped baby spinach

1 tablespoon Tridoshic Masala (page 179)

Chopped cilantro leaf, for garnish

Shredded coconut, for garnish (optional; omit for Kapha)

### To make the dal

1. Put the water, mung dal, and coconut oil into a stovetop pressure cooker and stir well.

2. Cover the pan and cook over high heat for 5 to 6 minutes, or until the cooker whistles.

3. Reduce the heat to medium-low and cook for 3 minutes more.

4. Turn off the burner but keep the pressure cooker on the warm burner. Allow the pressure to release naturally before opening. The consistency of the dal should be thick, soft, creamy, and smooth.

### To make the sambar

1. In a medium saucepan, heat the coconut oil over medium-low heat. Add the onion, cumin seeds, and brown mustard seeds. Sauté for 2 minutes, stirring frequently.

2. Add the black pepper, ¼ teaspoon of salt, turmeric, cayenne pepper (if using), serrano pepper, ginger, and curry leaves. Sauté for 1 minute, stirring constantly.

3. Add 3 cups of water and bring to a boil.

4. Reduce the boiling water to medium, and add the beets, yellow squash, and carrots. Cook, mostly covered, for 5 minutes.

5. Put the tamarind paste in ⅓ cup of warm water. Stir well until dissolved and set aside.

6. After the veggies have been cooking for 5 minutes, add the spinach and stir well.

7. Reduce the heat to a low simmer. Add the tamarind mixture, Tridoshic Masala, and the remaining ¼ teaspoon of salt. Stir well.

8. Add the cooked dal and stir thoroughly. The sambar should become slightly thick and creamy.

9. Simmer the sambar for an additional 3 to 5 minutes.

10. Garnish with a handful of cilantro and a sprinkle of coconut (if using).

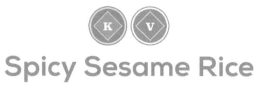

# Spicy Sesame Rice

**SERVES 5 TO 6 / PREP TIME: 5 MINUTES / COOK TIME: 15 MINUTES**

Here's a flavorful twist on everyday basmati rice. The seasoning makes it detoxifying and an ideal choice for cleansing, illness, and weak digestion. Although plain basmati rice has Kapha-provoking properties, the powerful blend of spices in this recipe balances out the cooling, sticky, heavy nature of the rice, making it suitable for Kapha types.

**For the rice**

2 cups water

1 cup basmati rice

2 teaspoons ghee, divided

**For the seasoning**

3 tablespoons sesame seeds
(use 2 tablespoons for Kapha)

2 teaspoons black peppercorns, whole

1 tablespoon cumin seeds, whole

1½ teaspoons brown mustard
seeds, whole

**To make the rice**

1. In a medium saucepan, bring the water to a boil.

2. Rinse the basmati rice under warm water. Strain and set aside.

3. Once the water is boiling, reduce the heat to low and add the basmati rice and 1 teaspoon of ghee. Stir well.

4. Cook, mostly covered, for 12 minutes. Cover with the lid completely around 6 minutes.

5. Turn off the heat, but leave the pan on the hot burner. Add the remaining 1 teaspoon of ghee and stir well. Cover the pan and let sit for 5 minutes.

**To make the seasoning**

1. Put the sesame seeds, black peppercorns, cumin seeds, and brown mustard seeds in a spice grinder or blender, and grind them until the mixture is powdered.

2. Heat a small sauté pan or skillet over medium heat.

3. In the heated pan, dry roast the powdered spice blend for 2 to 3 minutes, stirring frequently.

4. Add the roasted spices to the cooked rice, and stir well until the rice is evenly coated.

5. Serve this rice as a spicy base to any dal recipe, or top it with any vegetable or curry dish.

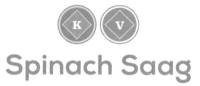

# Spinach Saag

GOOD FOR: Anemia, High Blood Pressure, Bone Health, Complexion, Weight Loss, Inflammation, Cancer Prevention, Pregnancy, Postpartum

**SERVES 4 TO 5 / PREP TIME: 10 TO 15 MINUTES / COOK TIME: 10 MINUTES**

Here is a traditional Indian dish that is as tasty as it is nutritious! Spinach Saag can help build your blood and strengthen your bones, and also promotes weight loss and heart health.

3 tablespoons ghee

½ medium onion, chopped

½ teaspoon brown mustard seeds, whole

½ teaspoon cumin seeds, whole

¼ teaspoon salt, divided

4 garlic cloves, finely chopped

2-inch piece fresh ginger, minced

1 teaspoon turmeric powder

⅛ to ¼ teaspoon cayenne pepper (optional)

1 teaspoon Vata Masala (page 178)

¼ cup water

16 ounces baby spinach

¼ cup chopped cilantro leaves

Juice of ½ lime

1. In a large sauté pan or skillet, heat the ghee over medium heat.

2. Add the onion, brown mustard seeds, cumin seeds, and ⅛ teaspoon of salt. Cook over medium heat for 2 minutes, stirring frequently.

3. Add the garlic and ginger. Cook for 2 minutes, stirring frequently.

4. Add the turmeric, cayenne pepper (if using), and Vata Masala. Stirring constantly, cook for 30 seconds.

5. Add the water and chopped spinach. Stirring constantly, cook for 5 minutes, or until the spinach has wilted and turned a bright green.

6. Turn the heat off, but keep the pan on the hot burner. Add the cilantro, lime juice, and remaining ⅛ teaspoon of salt. Stir well.

7. Enjoy over Everyday Basmati Rice (page 92) or Spicy Sesame Rice (page 114).

# Curried Cauliflower, Potato, and Kale Subji

**GOOD FOR:** Digestion, Constipation, Anemia, Energy, Weight Loss, Colon Health, Heart Health, Liver Health, Cancer Prevention

**SERVES 4 TO 6 / PREP TIME: 15 MINUTES / COOK TIME: 15 MINUTES**

*Subji* means "vegetable" and is often included as a side dish to dal, rice, and chapati. This curried subji uses a deliciously healing blend of cauliflower, potato, and kale, making it a solid choice to address heart health, liver health, colon health, weight loss, and iron deficiency.

### For the sauce

1 cup water

½ teaspoon chopped serrano pepper

¼ cup chopped cilantro

2 tablespoons coarsely chopped ginger

1 teaspoon turmeric powder

¾ teaspoon cumin powder

¼ teaspoon salt

2 tablespoons shredded coconut (use 1 tablespoon for Kapha)

2 tablespoons coconut oil (use 1 tablespoon for Kapha)

⅛ teaspoon cayenne pepper (omit for Pitta)

Juice of 1 lime

### For the sauté

1 tablespoon coconut oil

½ teaspoon cumin seeds, whole

½ teaspoon brown mustard seeds, whole

¼ teaspoon freshly ground black pepper

½ cup minced onion

2½ cups chopped cauliflower

1½ cups chopped potato

¼ cup water

2 cups stemmed and chopped kale

2 tablespoons finely minced cilantro

1 tablespoon shredded coconut

¼ teaspoon salt

continued ▶

**To make the sauce**

1. Combine the water, serrano pepper, cilantro, ginger, turmeric, cumin, salt, shredded coconut, coconut oil, cayenne pepper (if using), and lime juice to a blender.

2. Blend on high for 1 to 3 minutes until a thick, smooth liquid has formed. Set aside.

**To make the sauté**

1. In a large, deep sauté pan or skillet, heat the coconut oil over medium heat.

2. Add the cumin seeds, brown mustard seeds, black pepper, and onion. Sauté uncovered for 3 minutes, stirring frequently.

3. Add the cauliflower, potato, and water. Continue to sauté uncovered for 3 minutes, stirring frequently.

4. Add the prepared sauce and kale. Cover the pan and increase the heat slightly to medium-high. Cook for 3 minutes, stirring at the halfway point.

5. Uncover the pan and continue to cook for 6 minutes more, stirring every 2 to 3 minutes.

6. Turn the heat off, but leave the pan on the hot burner. Add the cilantro, coconut, and salt. Stir well.

7. Serve as a side dish to any savory meal, or enjoy this subji on its own as a light, healthy lunch or dinner. This recipe is most balancing when eaten in the winter and spring seasons.

# Sautéed Kale and Golden Tahini Sauce

**GOOD FOR:** Digestion, Constipation, Anemia, Bone Health, Colon Health, Heart Health, Liver Health, Cancer Prevention

**SERVES 4 TO 5 / PREP TIME: 15 MINUTES / COOK TIME: 15 MINUTES**

Because of kale's bitter, dry, cooling, and rough qualities, it increases Vata and can provoke symptoms like gas, bloating, dryness, spaciness, and anxiety. Luckily, with the proper complementary ingredients, you can balance these qualities and make it suitable for Vata types.

1 bunch green kale, stemmed

1 tablespoon sesame oil

½ teaspoon cumin seeds, whole

¼ teaspoon brown mustard seeds, whole

⅛ teaspoon freshly ground black pepper

Large pinch cayenne pepper (optional)

¼ cup water

¾ cup Golden Tahini Sauce (page 184)

⅛ teaspoon salt

Juice of ¼ lemon

1. Chop the kale leaves into thin strips, about ¼ to ½ inch in thickness. Set aside.

2. In a large sauté pan or skillet, heat the sesame oil over medium heat. Add the cumin seeds, brown mustard seeds, and black pepper. Sauté for 2 minutes, stirring frequently. Add the cayenne pepper (if using) and sauté for 30 seconds.

3. Stir in the chopped kale and the water. Sauté over medium heat, uncovered, for 5 to 7 minutes or until the kale is bright green, moist, and tender.

4. Take the pan off the heat. Add the tahini sauce and stir until the kale is evenly coated.

5. Add the salt and lemon juice. Combine well and serve.

6. Eat, share, and nourish.

# Colorful Quinoa Salad

**GOOD FOR:** Energy, Weight Loss, Anemia, Eye Health, Skin Health, Heart Health, Immunity, Pregnancy

**SERVES 4 TO 6 / PREP TIME: 10 MINUTES / COOK TIME: 20 MINUTES
(PLUS 30 MINUTES TO SOAK, OPTIONAL)**

This irresistible salad uses chilled quinoa and colorful vegetables to create a vibrant, delicious meal to enjoy throughout the spring and summer seasons. This salad is best for Kapha and Pitta types, but can be made Vata-friendly with a few simple modifications (see Health Tip).

**For the quinoa**

2¼ cups water

1 cup uncooked quinoa

½ teaspoon salt

1 tablespoon olive oil

**For the salad**

1 tablespoon olive oil

½ teaspoon cumin seeds, whole

¼ teaspoon brown mustard seeds, whole (omit for Pitta)

⅛ teaspoon freshly ground black pepper

⅓ cup raw pumpkin seeds

¼ teaspoon salt, divided

⅓ cup chopped red bell pepper

⅓ cup chopped orange bell pepper

⅓ cup chopped yellow squash

⅓ cup chopped zucchini

2 tablespoons balsamic vinegar (use 1 tablespoon for Pitta)

Juice of 1 lime

¼ cup minced cilantro

Avocado, cubed (optional)

**To prepare the quinoa**

1. If time permits, soak the quinoa for 30 minutes in warm water prior to cooking. Drain and discard the water (optional).

2. In a medium saucepan, bring the water to a boil.

**3.** Add the quinoa, salt, and olive oil, and reduce the heat to medium-low. Cook, mostly covered, for 13 minutes, stirring at the halfway point.

**4.** Turn off the heat, but keep the pan on the hot burner. Completely cover the pan, and let the quinoa sit for an additional 5 minutes.

**5.** Put the quinoa in a large salad or mixing bowl and refrigerate, uncovered, to allow the quinoa to cool.

**To prepare the salad**

**1.** In a medium sauté pan or skillet, heat the olive oil over medium heat.

**2.** Add the cumin seeds, brown mustard seeds, and black pepper and sauté for 1 minute, stirring frequently.

**3.** Add the pumpkin seeds and ⅛ teaspoon of salt. Continue to sauté for 2 minutes, stirring frequently.

**4.** Add the red and orange bell peppers, yellow squash, and zucchini. Sauté for 1 to 2 minutes more, stirring constantly.

**5.** Take the quinoa out of the refrigerator and add the sautéed ingredients. Stir well to ensure even blending.

**6.** Add the balsamic vinegar, the remaining ⅛ teaspoon of salt, lime juice, and cilantro. Stir well.

**7.** Top each serving with the avocado (if using). If more protein is needed, top with Roasted Zucchini Tahini Hummus (page 99), or any hummus you prefer.

**+ HEALTH TIP:**

*Make this salad Vata-balancing by replacing the bell peppers with some more suitable, Vata-reducing veggies such as asparagus, spinach, peas, artichokes, olives, or carrots.*

# Summertime Salad

**GOOD FOR:** Energy, Weight Loss, Excessive Heat, Colon Health, Heart Health, Cancer Prevention

**SERVES 2 / PREP TIME: 15 MINUTES**

This delicious salad features a variety of seasonal, colorful vegetables paired with digestion-enhancing ingredients. Pitta and Kapha types can eat this throughout the summer, and it is also suitable for Vata types on occasion.

4 cups chopped butter leaf or romaine lettuce

2 cups chopped baby spinach

6 artichoke hearts, chopped

8 kalamata olives, pitted and chopped (omit for Pitta)

6 cucumber slices, quartered

⅓ cup chopped red pepper

1 avocado, cubed (omit for Kapha)

1 tablespoon sunflower seeds

2 tablespoons olive oil

2 tablespoons fresh lemon juice (use lime for Pitta)

⅛ teaspoon salt

Pinch freshly ground black pepper

2 cups hummus, divided

½ cup sprouts, divided (omit for Vata)

1. In a large mixing bowl, combine the lettuce, spinach, artichoke hearts, olives, cucumber, and red pepper.

2. Add the avocado and sunflower seeds.

3. In a small bowl, combine the olive oil, lemon juice, salt, and black pepper. Stir well and pour over the salad mixture. Toss the salad until all the ingredients have been evenly blended.

4. Serve the salad on plates.

5. Top each salad with 1 cup of hummus and ⅛ cup of sprouts. For the hummus, use Roasted Zucchini Tahini Hummus (page 99), Coconut Curry Hummus (page 98), or any store-bought variety you enjoy.

# Simply Delicious Lettuce Wrap

**GOOD FOR:** Digestion, Energy, Weight Loss, Excessive Heat, Colon Health, Heart Health

**SERVES 2 / PREP TIME: 10 MINUTES**

These light, simple, cooling wraps are a summertime essential for keeping healthy, happy, and balanced. Even Vata types can enjoy these summertime wraps on occasion; just omit the sprouts, add a drizzle of olive oil, use extra avocado, and add a splash of lemon.

6 large leaves butter leaf lettuce

1½ cups hummus

12 cucumber slices

4 roma tomatoes, sliced

1½ cups sprouts, divided

1 avocado, cubed
(optional; omit for Kapha)

Balsamic vinegar
(optional; omit for Pitta)

1. Rinse the lettuce and dry thoroughly. Lay each leaf flat on a plate.

2. Spread ¼ cup of hummus vertically down the center of each leaf. Use Roasted Zucchini Tahini Hummus (page 99), Coconut Curry Hummus (page 98), or any store-bought variety you enjoy.

3. Place 2 cucumber slices lengthwise on top of the hummus.

4. Place 2 or 3 tomato slices on top of the cucumber. (Pittas should reduce this amount to 1 slice per wrap.)

5. Spread ¼ cup of sprouts on top of the tomato.

6. Top each wrap with a few avocado cubes (if using) and a drizzle of balsamic vinegar (if using).

7. Roll the edges up to make a secure wrap. If available, place a toothpick in the center to hold the wrap. Enjoy!

**INGREDIENT TIP:**

*Pitta types can substitute an Essential Chapati (page 93) wrap in place of the lettuce leaf, and Kapha types can try a collard green leaf to add even more flavor and nutrients.*

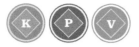

# Simply Steamed Veggies

**SERVES 2 TO 4 / PREP TIME: 10 MINUTES / COOK TIME: 15 MINUTES**

This quick and easy recipe requires only a handful of accessible, affordable ingredients. These steamed veggies support you in healing digestion, promoting healthy elimination, enhancing overall nutrition, and strengthening your mind.

1 medium zucchini, chopped small

1 medium yellow squash, chopped small

1 cup chopped cauliflower

1 small carrot, thinly sliced

1 cup chopped broccoli

1 tablespoon ghee

¼ teaspoon salt

Large pinch freshly ground black pepper

1. Fill a large saucepan with 2 inches of water. Place a steamer basket in the pan. Turn the heat to high. If the water boils before the vegetables are chopped, reduce the heat to low and cover the pan.

2. Place the zucchini, yellow squash, cauliflower, carrot, and broccoli into the steamer basket.

3. Set the heat to medium-low and cook, mostly covered, for 12 minutes.

4. Check on your veggies at 12 minutes. They should be vibrant in color and slightly soft all the way through. If they are still too raw, cover the pan and cook for 5 minutes more, checking every minute to avoid oversteaming.

5. When the veggies are done, transfer them to a large bowl.

6. Add the ghee, salt, and black pepper.

7. Stir the ingredients together until the ghee evenly coats all the veggies.

8. Serve, sit, and enjoy! These steamed veggies can be eaten as a healthy snack, tasty side dish, or a light dinner.

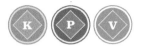

# Curried Coconut and Veggie Soup

**GOOD FOR:** Energy, Digestion, Constipation, Eye Health, Skin Health, Heart Health, Colon Health, Cancer Prevention, Immunity, Pregnancy, Postpartum

**SERVES 5 TO 6 / PREP TIME: 15 MINUTES / COOK TIME: 15 MINUTES**

This puréed soup makes a creamy, vibrant meal that is packed with flavor. By steaming the vegetables, you preserve their vitamin and mineral content, increase their sweetness, and make them more digestible for your system.

3 cups chopped sweet potato

2 cups chopped zucchini

1 cup chopped cauliflower

2 tablespoons coconut oil, divided (cut the amount in half for Kapha)

½ teaspoon cumin seeds, whole

¼ teaspoon freshly ground black pepper

⅛ teaspoon cayenne pepper (optional; omit for Pitta)

½ cup water

2 cups coconut water (use 2 cups plain water for Kapha)

5 tablespoons pumpkin seeds

2 tablespoons shredded coconut (use 1 tablespoon for Kapha)

1½ teaspoons Tridoshic Masala (page 179)

1 teaspoon ground cinnamon

⅛ teaspoon cardamom powder

Fresh ginger (2-inch cube), chopped

½ teaspoon salt

**1.** Fill a large saucepan with 2 inches of water. Place a steamer basket in the pan. Turn the heat to high. If the water boils before the vegetables are chopped, reduce the heat to low and cover the pan.

**2.** Place the sweet potato, zucchini, and cauliflower into the steamer basket.

**3.** Set the heat to medium-low and cook, mostly covered, for 12 minutes. The vegetables should be vibrant in color and slightly soft all the way through. If they are still too raw, cook for 1 to 5 minutes more, checking every minute.

continued ▶

4. When the veggies are done, transfer them to a large bowl. Do not keep them in the pan, because they will overcook.

5. In a small sauté pan or skillet, heat 1 tablespoon of coconut oil over medium heat. Add the cumin seeds and black pepper, and sauté for 1 to 2 minutes, stirring occasionally.

6. Add the cayenne pepper (if using) and sauté for 30 seconds more, stirring continuously. Set aside until needed.

7. Pour the water and coconut water into a blender.

8. Add to the blender the sautéed spices, remaining 1 tablespoon of coconut oil, pumpkin seeds, shredded coconut, Tridoshic Masala, cinnamon, cardamom, ginger, and salt.

9. Blend on high for 1 to 3 minutes, or until a thick, creamy, and smooth consistency has been reached.

10. Add the steamed vegetables and blend for 2 to 3 minutes, or until a smooth and creamy texture has been reached.

11. Serve in small bowls and garnish with some shredded coconut, salt, pepper, and coconut oil if desired.

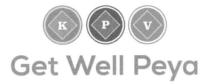

# Get Well Peya

**GOOD FOR:** Digestion, Detox, Constipation, Congestion, Illness, Immunity, Weight Loss, Postpartum

**SERVES 4 TO 6 / PREP TIME: 5 MINUTES / COOK TIME: 25 MINUTES**

Peya is a soupy rice recipe that is often part of a cleanse. The digestive, detoxifying spices aid the cleansing process and help to flush the toxins (*ama*) from your system while increasing the digestive fire (*agni*).

1 cup basmati rice

2 tablespoons ghee

½ teaspoon cumin seeds, whole

½ teaspoon freshly ground black pepper

2 tablespoons minced onion

1 or 2 cloves garlic, finely minced

8 cups water

1 teaspoon ground ginger or finely grated fresh ginger

¼ teaspoon turmeric powder

Large pinch cayenne pepper (optional)

¼ teaspoon salt

Chopped cilantro, for garnish

Chopped scallions (green parts), for garnish (optional)

Pinch freshly ground black pepper

1. Rinse the basmati rice under warm water. Strain and set aside.

2. In an open stovetop pressure cooker, heat the ghee over medium heat. Add the cumin seeds, black pepper, onion, and garlic. Sauté for 2 minutes, stirring frequently.

3. To the pressure cooker, add the water, rice, ginger, turmeric, cayenne pepper (if using), and salt. Stir well.

4. Secure the lid on the pressure cooker. Heat on high heat for 5 to 6 minutes, or until the pressure cooker begins to whistle.

5. Reduce the heat to medium-low and cook for 10 minutes.

continued ▷

6. Turn the heat off, but leave the pan on the hot burner. Allow the pressure to release naturally, waiting at least 10 to 15 minutes before opening the lid.

7. Open the lid and stir the rice. You should have a thick, liquid rice soup, similar to a porridge.

8. Serve in a bowl and top with cilantro, scallions (if using), and black pepper. More salt can be added if needed. During a cleanse, more ghee can be added as well.

9. Peya is best fresh; however, it will last for 2 to 3 days in the refrigerator. When reheating, add a splash of water, fresh ghee, and a dash of black pepper.

## + HEALTH TIP:

*Eat one bowl of this soup 3 to 6 times a day during sickness, cleansing, weakness, digestion disturbances, and directly after giving birth. To maintain digestive health, Vata types can perform a Peya fast one day each month, Pitta types one day every two weeks, and Kapha types one day each week. Complement this fast with the Detox Tonic (page 52).*

Spicy Red Lentil Dal and Everyday Basmati Rice 92 and 144

# DINNERS

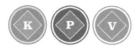

# Classic Cleansing Kitchari

**GOOD FOR:** Digestion, Detox, Weight Loss, Colon Health, Liver Health, Pregnancy, Postpartum

**SERVES 5 TO 6 / PREP TIME: 5 MINUTES / COOK TIME: 25 MINUTES**

Kitchari is a staple for an Ayurvedic diet and essential for an Ayurvedic cleanse. This tridoshic kitchari recipe provides healing during times of digestive issues, constipation, illness, weakness, and flu. It gives your digestion a break after indulging a bit too much, and helps strengthen your digestive fire while flushing out any built-up toxins.

2 tablespoons ghee

¼ cup minced onion

½ teaspoon cumin seeds, whole

½ teaspoon brown mustard seeds, whole (omit for Pitta)

½ teaspoon freshly ground black pepper

2 tablespoons finely minced fresh ginger

1 teaspoon finely minced serrano pepper (optional; omit for Pitta)

⅛ teaspoon cayenne pepper (optional; omit for Pitta)

2 teaspoons Tridoshic Masala (page 179)

6 cups water

1 cup split mung dal

¾ cup basmati rice (use quinoa for Kapha)

⅓ cup thinly sliced carrot

½ cup thinly sliced celery

1 cup chopped kale leaves, stemmed

¼ cup finely chopped cilantro

Juice of ½ lemon (use lime for Pitta)

¾ teaspoon salt

Lemon wedges, for garnish (use lime for Pitta)

Chopped scallions (green parts), for garnish

Ghee, for serving

1. In a large saucepan, heat the ghee over medium heat. Add the onion, cumin seeds, brown mustard seeds, and black pepper, and sauté for 2 minutes.

2. Add the ginger, serrano pepper (if using), cayenne pepper (if using), and Tridoshic Masala. Sauté for 30 seconds, stirring constantly.

3. Add the water and bring to a boil over high heat.

4. Once boiling, reduce the heat to medium and add the mung dal. Cook, mostly covered, for 10 minutes, stirring at the halfway point.

5. After 10 minutes, add the rice, carrot, celery, and kale. Stir well. Cook, mostly covered, over medium-low heat for 12 minutes, stirring every 3 to 4 minutes. If the kitchari becomes too thick, add a little more water.

6. After 12 minutes, reduce the heat to low, cover the pan completely, and cook for 3 minutes more. Stir every minute.

7. Turn off the heat and take the pan off the hot burner. Add the cilantro, lemon juice, and salt. Stir well. Cover the pan and let sit for a few minutes to allow the flavors to harmonize.

8. Garnish with lemon wedges and scallions and serve.

9. For added cleansing effects, top each serving generously with extra cilantro, lemon juice (lime for Pitta), and ghee. Add more salt and pepper if needed.

# Kapha-Reducing Kitchari

**GOOD FOR:** Digestion, Detox, Weight Loss, Energy, Allergies, Congestion, Circulation, Heart Health, Blood Sugar Balance, High Cholesterol, Pregnancy, Postpartum

**SERVES 4 TO 5 / PREP TIME: 5 MINUTES / COOK TIME: 25 MINUTES**

This light, easy-to-digest kitchari recipe was created specifically for kindling the digestive fire, removing toxins, and balancing excessive Kapha in the system. The stimulating spices are sure to boost your energy, metabolism, and mood, while leaving you light and ready to go!

1 tablespoon sunflower oil

¼ cup minced onion

½ teaspoon cumin seeds, whole

½ teaspoon brown mustard seeds, whole

¼ teaspoon freshly ground black pepper

2 cloves garlic, finely minced

2 teaspoons Kapha Masala (page 176)

1 teaspoon ground ginger

⅛ teaspoon cayenne pepper

5½ cups water

1 cup mung dal

½ cup quinoa

1 medium carrot, thinly sliced

2 celery stalks, thinly sliced

1 cup chopped cauliflower

½ cup chopped broccoli

2 cups chopped baby spinach

Juice of 1 lemon

½ teaspoon pink Himalayan salt

Chopped cilantro, for garnish

Chopped scallions (green parts), for garnish

1. In a large saucepan, warm the sunflower oil over medium heat. Add the onion, cumin seeds, brown mustard seeds, and black pepper. Sauté for 2 minutes, stirring frequently.

2. Add the garlic, Kapha Masala, ginger, and cayenne. Sauté for 30 seconds, stirring constantly.

3. Add the water and bring to a boil.

4. Reduce the heat to medium and add the mung dal. Stir well and cook, mostly covered, for 10 minutes, stirring at the halfway point.

5. Add the quinoa, carrot, celery, cauliflower, and broccoli. Stir well. Cook, mostly covered, over medium-low heat for 10 minutes, stirring every 3 to 4 minutes. If the kitchari becomes too thick, add a little more water.

6. Add the spinach, reduce the heat to low, cover the pan completely, and cook for 5 minutes. Stir every minute.

7. Turn off the heat, but leave the pan on the hot burner. Add the lemon juice and salt. Stir well. Cover the pan and let sit for a few minutes to allow the flavors to harmonize.

8. Serve into individual bowls. Garnish generously with cilantro, scallions, and additional lemon juice and black pepper if desired.

# Pitta-Reducing Kitchari

**GOOD FOR:** Digestion, Detox, Inflammation, Excessive Heat, Complexion, Eczema, Hyperacidity, Colon Health, Liver Health, Pregnancy, Postpartum

**SERVES 5 TO 6 / PREP TIME: 5 MINUTES / COOK TIME: 25 MINUTES**

This kitchari uses only cooling, Pitta-soothing ingredients such as ghee, coconut, cilantro, lime, kale, celery, zucchini, and Pitta Masala. Together with the mung dal and basmati rice, this recipe is sure to cool off any excessive heat, soothe inflammation, and keep your Pitta in balance, no matter the time of year.

2 tablespoons ghee

1 teaspoon cumin seeds, whole

⅛ teaspoon freshly ground black pepper

1½ teaspoons Pitta Masala (page 177)

2 tablespoons finely minced fresh ginger

2 tablespoons shredded coconut

6 cups water

1 cup mung dal

¾ cup basmati rice

½ cup chopped zucchini

½ cup chopped yellow squash

5 asparagus stalks, chopped

1 large celery stick, thinly sliced

1 large kale leaf, stemmed and thinly sliced

½ cup cilantro, finely chopped, plus for garnish

Juice of 1 lime

½ teaspoon pink Himalayan salt

Shredded coconut, for garnish

Ghee, for individual servings

1. In a large saucepan, heat the ghee over medium heat. Add the cumin and black pepper. Sauté for 2 minutes, stirring frequently.

2. Add the Pitta Masala, ginger, and coconut. Stirring constantly, sauté for 30 seconds more.

3. Add the water and bring the mixture to a boil.

4. Add the mung dal and reduce the heat to medium. Cook, mostly covered, for 10 minutes, stirring at the halfway point.

5. Add the rice, zucchini, yellow squash, asparagus, celery, and kale. Stir well. Reduce the heat slightly to medium-low and cook, mostly covered, for 12 minutes.

6. Stir every 3 to 4 minutes during the remaining cooking time. If the kitchari becomes too thick, add a little more water.

7. Reduce the heat to low, cover the pan completely, and cook for 3 minutes, stirring at the halfway point.

8. Turn off the heat, and take the pan off the hot burner. Add the cilantro, lime juice, and salt. Stir well, cover, and let sit for 3 minutes to let all the flavors soak in.

9. Garnish each bowl with extra cilantro, shredded coconut, and ghee. Add any additional lime juice, salt, and black pepper if needed.

10. Take a deep breath, sit comfortably in a peaceful space, and enjoy with good company!

# Vata-Reducing Kitchari

**GOOD FOR:** Digestion, Detox, Constipation, Energy, Circulation, Anemia, Anxiety, Insomnia, Pregnancy, Postpartum, Lactation

**SERVES 4 TO 6 / PREP TIME: 5 MINUTES / COOK TIME: 25 MINUTES**

This grounding kitchari recipe is an excellent meal for fall and winter months. Vata types need three warm, well-cooked, nourishing meals daily, and this recipe makes a wonderful addition.

2 tablespoons sesame oil

¼ cup minced onion

½ teaspoon cumin seeds, whole

½ teaspoon brown mustard seeds, whole

¼ teaspoon freshly ground black pepper

1 teaspoon Vata Masala (page 178)

2 tablespoons finely minced fresh ginger

2 tablespoons shredded coconut

⅛ teaspoon cayenne pepper

7 cups bone, chicken, or vegetable broth (or substitute water)

2 cinnamon sticks

1 cup mung dal

1 cup basmati rice

1 medium carrot, thinly sliced

½ cup chopped sweet potato

⅓ cup chopped beet

½ cup chopped cauliflower

2 cups baby spinach, chopped

Juice of 1 lemon

½ teaspoon pink Himalayan salt

Ghee, for serving

Chopped cilantro, for garnish

Shredded coconut, for garnish

1. In a large saucepan, heat the sesame oil over medium heat. Add the onion, cumin, brown mustard seeds, and black pepper. Sauté for 2 minutes, stirring frequently.

2. Add the Vata Masala, ginger, coconut, and cayenne. Sauté for 30 seconds, stirring constantly.

3. Add the broth and cinnamon sticks and bring to a boil.

4. Add the mung dal and cook, mostly covered, over medium heat for 10 minutes, stirring at the halfway point.

5. Add the rice, carrot, sweet potato, beet, and cauliflower. Stir well. Cook, mostly covered, for 10 minutes, stirring every 3 to 4 minutes.

6. Add the spinach, reduce the heat to low, cover the pan completely, and cook for 5 minutes. Stir every 1 to 2 minutes.

7. Turn off the heat, but leave the pan on the hot burner. Add the lemon juice and salt. Stir well. Cover the pan and let sit for a few minutes to allow the flavors to harmonize.

8. Serve into bowls. For added Vata-reducing effects, add 1 teaspoon of ghee per serving and garnish generously with cilantro and coconut. More lemon juice, salt, and pepper can be added if needed.

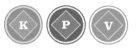

# Tridoshic Mung Dal and Quinoa Kitchari

**GOOD FOR:** Digestion, Detox, Weight Loss, Energy, Bone Health, Blood Sugar Balance, Heart Health, Constipation, Pregnancy, Postpartum

**SERVES 4 TO 6 / PREP TIME: 5 MINUTES / COOK TIME: 25 MINUTES**

This balanced kitchari recipe uses quinoa rather than basmati rice, which can be too sticky and heavy for some people (especially Kapha types). The colorful veggies provide a cleansing, alkalizing, and nutritive effect, and the gently warming digestive spices benefit all doshas.

1 tablespoon sesame oil (use coconut oil for Pitta)

½ teaspoon cumin seeds, whole

¼ teaspoon freshly ground black pepper

½ teaspoon turmeric powder

1 teaspoon Tridoshic Masala (page 179)

1 tablespoon finely grated fresh ginger

1 tablespoon shredded coconut (omit for Kapha)

6½ cups water

1 cup mung dal

1 cup quinoa

½ medium zucchini, chopped

½ medium yellow squash, chopped

1 celery stalk, thinly sliced

1 medium carrot, thinly sliced

1 cup chopped baby spinach (use kale for Pitta)

½ teaspoon pink Himalayan salt

Juice of 1 lime

Chopped cilantro leaves, for garnish

Chopped scallions (green parts), for garnish

Shredded coconut, for garnish (omit for Kapha)

Ghee, for serving (optional)

1. In a large saucepan, heat the sesame oil over medium heat. Add the cumin seeds and black pepper. Sauté for 2 minutes, stirring frequently.

2. Add the turmeric, Tridoshic Masala, ginger, and coconut. Sauté for 30 seconds, stirring continuously.

3. Add the water and bring to a boil.

4. Add the mung dal and cook, mostly covered, over medium heat for 10 minutes, stirring at the halfway point.

5. Add the quinoa, zucchini, yellow squash, celery, and carrot. Cook, mostly covered, on medium heat for 10 minutes. Stir every 3 to 4 minutes. If the kitchari becomes too thick, add a little more water.

6. Add the spinach, reduce the heat to low, cover the pan completely, and cook for 5 minutes. Stir every 1 to 2 minutes.

7. Check on the dal to make sure it is soft, mushy, and well-cooked. The veggies should be soft, but still vibrant in color.

8. Turn off the heat. Add the salt and lime juice. Blend well. Cover the pan and let sit for 3 minutes to allow the flavors to come together.

9. Top each bowl with cilantro, scallions, and coconut. Add 1 teaspoon of ghee (if using) per serving.

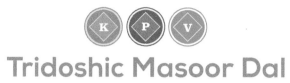

# Tridoshic Masoor Dal

**GOOD FOR:** Digestion, Detox, Constipation, Energy, Hair Health, Skin Health, Heart Health, Colon Health, Immunity, Pregnancy, Postpartum

**SERVES 5 TO 6 / PREP TIME: 5 MINUTES / COOK TIME: 25 MINUTES**

This red lentil (masoor) dal recipe is healing for all body types and can be enjoyed anytime of year. Masoor dal is delicious when served over basmati rice, and tastes just as yummy when eaten with brown rice, quinoa, millet, or a chapati.

2 tablespoons ghee

¼ cup minced onion

½ teaspoon cumin seeds, whole

½ teaspoon brown mustard seeds, whole (omit for Pitta)

¼ teaspoon freshly ground black pepper

2 tablespoons finely minced fresh ginger

1 tablespoon shredded coconut (Omit for Kapha)

2 teaspoons Tridoshic Masala (page 179)

⅛ teaspoon cayenne pepper (optional; omit for Pitta)

6 cups water

2 cups red lentils (masoor dal)

½ cup thinly sliced carrots

1 cup thinly sliced celery

½ cup chopped cauliflower

2 cups chopped baby spinach (use kale for Pitta)

Juice of 1 lime

½ teaspoon salt

Finely chopped cilantro, for garnish

Shredded coconut, for garnish (omit for Kapha)

Chopped scallions (green parts), for garnish

1. In a large saucepan, heat the ghee over medium heat. Add the onion, cumin seeds, brown mustard seeds, and black pepper. Sauté for 2 minutes, stirring frequently.

2. Add ginger, coconut, Tridoshic Masala, and cayenne pepper (if using), and sauté for 30 seconds more, stirring constantly.

3. Add the water and bring to a boil.

4. Add the red lentils and stir well. Reduce the heat to medium and cook, mostly covered, for 5 minutes, stirring at the halfway point.

5. Add the carrots, celery, and cauliflower. Stir well and continue to cook for 10 minutes. Stir every 3 to 4 minutes.

6. Add the spinach and reduce the heat to a low simmer. Cook, mostly covered, for 5 minutes, stirring at the halfway point.

7. Take the pan off the heat, and add the lime juice and salt.

8. Top each serving with the cilantro, coconut, and scallions. Extra salt, pepper, and ghee can also be added as desired.

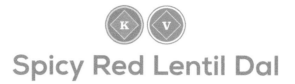

# Spicy Red Lentil Dal

**GOOD FOR:** Digestion, Detox, Constipation, Immunity, Energy, Anemia, Weight Loss, Heart Health, Circulation, Pregnancy, Postpartum

**SERVES 5 TO 6 / PREP TIME: 10 MINUTES / COOK TIME: 20 MINUTES**

The little red lentil makes an amazing addition to any diet: It cooks up quickly and is easy to digest. This spicy dal pairs wonderfully with Spicy Sesame Rice (page 114). Serve it with a generous spoonful of the Coconut-Cilantro Chutney (page 183).

1 tablespoon ghee

1 teaspoon cumin seeds, whole

1 teaspoon brown mustard seeds, whole

½ teaspoon fennel seeds, whole

¼ teaspoon freshly ground black pepper

¼ cup onion, minced

1 teaspoon turmeric powder

1 teaspoon ground ginger

Pinch hing (optional)

3 cloves garlic, finely minced

⅛ teaspoon cayenne pepper

1 medium jalapeño pepper, finely minced

6 cups water

2 cups red lentils (masoor dal)

1 medium carrot, thinly sliced

2 celery stalks, thinly sliced

3 kale leaves, stemmed and chopped (1½ cups chopped spinach for Vata)

¾ teaspoon salt

Juice of 1 lemon

Ghee, for serving (optional)

Chopped scallions (green parts), for garnish

Chopped cilantro leaves, for garnish

1. In a large saucepan, heat the ghee over medium heat. Add the cumin seeds, brown mustard seeds, fennel seeds, black pepper, and onion. Sauté for 2 minutes, stirring frequently.

2. Add the turmeric, ginger, hing (if using), garlic, cayenne pepper, and jalapeño pepper. Sauté for 30 seconds, stirring constantly.

3. Add the water and bring to a boil.

4. Reduce the heat to medium and add the red lentils. Cook, mostly covered, for 10 minutes.

5. Add the carrot, celery, and kale. Cook, mostly covered, over medium-low heat for 12 minutes more, stirring every 3 to 4 minutes. If the dal becomes too thick, add a little more water.

6. After 12 minutes, reduce the heat to low, cover the pan completely, and cook for 3 minutes, stirring every minute.

7. Take the pan off the heat. Add the salt and lemon juice. Stir well.

8. Serve over a bowl of rice, quinoa, or millet, or enjoy on its own. Garnish each bowl with ghee (if using), scallions, and cilantro. Add any additional lemon juice, salt, or pepper as desired.

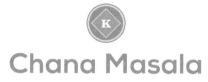

# Chana Masala

**GOOD FOR:** Digestion, Energy, Anemia, Weight Loss, Heart Health, Blood Sugar Balance, High Cholesterol, Circulation, Skin Health, Eye Health

**SERVES 4 / PREP TIME: 15 MINUTES / COOK TIME: 15 MINUTES**

A quintessential Kapha-reducing Indian dish, Chana Masala is flavorful and filling, yet light and energizing. It is traditionally served over basmati rice, although Kaphas will benefit most by enjoying it over a small bowl of quinoa, millet, or buckwheat—or by itself.

**For the curry sauce**

1 cup water

1 tablespoon coconut oil

½ cup chopped tomato

1 teaspoon chopped serrano pepper

Fresh ginger (2-inch cube), chopped

2 tablespoons shredded coconut

¼ cup chopped cilantro

Juice of ½ lime

⅛ teaspoon cayenne pepper

1 teaspoon Kapha Masala (page 176)

¼ teaspoon turmeric powder

½ teaspoon cumin seeds, whole

¼ teaspoon salt

**For the sauté**

1 tablespoon coconut oil

⅓ cup minced onion

½ teaspoon cumin seeds, whole

½ teaspoon brown mustard seeds, whole

¼ teaspoon freshly ground black pepper

1 tablespoon finely minced fresh ginger

1 cup chopped tomato

2 (15 ounce) cans chickpeas (3 cups cooked)

3 cups chopped baby spinach (5 ounces)

¼ cup chopped cilantro

Juice of ½ lime

¼ teaspoon salt

Chopped cilantro, for garnish

**To make the curry sauce**

1. Put the water, coconut oil, tomato, serrano pepper, ginger, coconut, cilantro, lime juice, cayenne pepper, Kapha Masala, turmeric, cumin seeds, and salt into a blender.

2. Blend on high for 1 to 2 minutes, or until everything is completely combined. Set aside.

**To make the sauté**

1. In a large, deep sauté pan or skillet, heat the coconut oil over medium heat. Add the onion, cumin seeds, brown mustard seeds, and black pepper. Sauté for 2 minutes, stirring frequently.

2. Add the ginger. Sauté for 1 minute more, stirring constantly.

3. Stir in the tomato, chickpeas, and curry sauce. Cover the pan and sauté over medium-high heat for 5 minutes. Stir every minute.

4. Reduce the heat to medium and stir in the spinach. Sauté uncovered for 5 to 7 minutes, stirring every minute.

5. Turn the heat off, but leave the pan on the hot burner. Add the cilantro, lime juice, and salt. Stir well.

6. Serve topped with cilantro.

**PAIRING TIP:**

*This spicy masala dish pairs delightfully with Spicy Sesame Rice (page 114) for even more heat, and Coconut-Cilantro Chutney (page 183) to cool things down.*

# Curried Black-Eyed Peas and Greens

**GOOD FOR:** Digestion, Energy, Inflammation, Anemia, Constipation, Weight Loss, Heart Health, Circulation, Skin Health, Eye Health, Pregnancy, Postpartum, Lactation

**SERVES 4 TO 5 / PREP TIME: 15 MINUTES / COOK TIME: 15 MINUTES**

Here you get a surprisingly flavorful black-eyed pea recipe that may just have you coming back for seconds! Although they can be Vata-provoking, the oil and spices in this recipe help alleviate the dry properties of this bean, allowing Vata types to enjoy this meal in moderation.

### For the curry sauce

¾ cup water

1 teaspoon chopped serrano pepper

1 tablespoon chopped fresh ginger

¼ cup chopped cilantro

Juice of 1 lime

⅛ teaspoon cayenne pepper (omit for Pitta)

1 teaspoon Kapha Masala (page 176)

½ teaspoon turmeric powder

¼ teaspoon salt

### For the sauté

2 tablespoons sunflower oil

½ cup minced onion (¼ cup for Pitta)

½ teaspoon cumin seeds, whole

½ teaspoon brown mustard seeds, whole (omit for Pitta)

¼ teaspoon freshly ground black pepper

2 tablespoons finely minced fresh ginger

1 clove garlic, finely minced

1 cup chopped kale leaf, stemmed

1 cup chopped collard greens, stemmed

3 cups chopped baby spinach

2 cans black-eyed peas (3 cups cooked)

3 scallions (white and green parts), chopped

¼ teaspoon salt

**To make the curry sauce**

1. Put the water, serrano pepper, ginger, cilantro, lime juice, cayenne pepper, Kapha Masala, turmeric, and salt into a blender.

2. Blend on high for 1 to 2 minutes or until everything is completely blended. Set aside until needed.

**To make the sauté**

1. In a large, deep sauté pan or skillet, warm the sunflower oil over medium heat. Add the onion, cumin seeds, brown mustard seeds, and black pepper. Sauté for 2 minutes, stirring frequently.

2. Add the ginger and garlic. Sauté for one minute, stirring constantly.

3. Stir in the kale, collard greens, and curry sauce. Sauté over medium heat, uncovered, for 5 minutes, stirring every minute.

4. Add the spinach, and continue to sauté for 3 minutes more, stirring every minute.

5. Add the black-eyed peas. Stir well and reduce the heat to medium-low. Cover the pan and cook for 3 minutes, stirring every minute.

6. Turn off the heat, and add the scallions and salt. Stir well.

7. Enjoy this dish on its own or over basmati rice, brown rice, quinoa, millet, or buckwheat.

# Chickpea and Kale Brown Rice Bowl

**GOOD FOR:** Digestion, Weight Loss, Constipation, Energy, Heart Health, Blood Sugar Balance, High Cholesterol, Pregnancy, Postpartum

**SERVES 4 / PREP TIME: 5 MINUTES / COOK TIME: 25 MINUTES**

The combination of chickpeas and brown rice in this bowl makes a complete protein. This healthy medley is equally rich in fiber, making it a great meal for appetite control, weight loss, digestion, and elimination.

---

**For the rice**

2 cups water

1 cup brown rice

1 tablespoon sunflower oil

⅛ teaspoon turmeric powder

1 cinnamon stick

⅛ teaspoon salt

1 tablespoon Spicy Stir-Fry Sauce (page 185)

**For the sauté**

1 tablespoon sunflower oil

⅓ cup minced onion

½ teaspoon cumin seeds, whole

½ teaspoon brown mustard seeds, whole

¼ teaspoon freshly ground black pepper

1 teaspoon Kapha Masala (page 176)

1 clove garlic, finely minced

Pinch cayenne pepper (optional)

2 tablespoons finely minced fresh ginger

4 kale leaves, stemmed and chopped

¼ cup water

2 (15-ounce) cans chickpeas (3 cups cooked)

¼ cup finely chopped cilantro, plus for garnish

2 tablespoons Spicy Stir-Fry Sauce (page 185)

**To make the rice**

1. Put the water, rice, sunflower oil, turmeric, cinnamon stick, and salt into a stovetop pressure cooker. Stir well and securely close the lid.

2. Set the heat to high and cook for 7 minutes, or until the cooker begins to whistle.

3. Reduce the heat to medium and continue to cook for 10 minutes.

4. Turn the heat off, but leave the pressure cooker on the hot burner. Let the cooker sit for 10 to 15 minutes.

5. Carefully open the lid. The rice should be moist and fluffy without any leftover liquid. Add 1 tablespoon of stir-fry sauce, cover, and set aside.

**To make the sauté**

1. In a large, deep sauté pan or skillet, heat the sunflower oil over medium heat. Add the onion, cumin seeds, brown mustard seeds, and black pepper. Sauté for 2 minutes, stirring frequently.

2. Add the Kapha Masala, garlic, cayenne pepper (if using), and ginger. Sauté for 30 seconds, stirring constantly.

3. Add the kale and water. Sauté for 2 minutes over medium heat, stirring frequently.

4. Add the chickpeas and continue to sauté for 2 to 3 minutes. The kale should be fully cooked with a vibrant green color and a moist, tender texture.

5. Turn off the heat. Add the cooked brown rice and blend all the ingredients together.

6. Add 2 tablespoons of stir-fry sauce. Stir well.

7. Serve in bowls, garnished with cilantro. Season to taste.

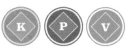

# Tridoshic Quinoa and Veggie Stir-Fry

**GOOD FOR:** Digestion, Constipation, Energy, Weight Loss, Inflammation, Heart Health, Colon Health, Cancer Prevention, Pregnancy, Postpartum

**SERVES 6 TO 8 / PREP TIME: 5 MINUTES / COOK TIME: 25 MINUTES**

This light and lovely dish will likely become your summertime favorite. Quinoa paired with a rainbow of fresh seasonal veggies delivers powerful antiaging benefits. This tridoshic stir-fry is best during the spring and summer seasons, but it is so delicious, you'll crave it year-round!

**For the quinoa**

4 cups water

2 cups quinoa

1 tablespoon coconut oil

¼ teaspoon turmeric

¼ teaspoon salt

**For the stir-fry**

2 tablespoons coconut oil

½ teaspoon cumin seeds, whole

½ teaspoon brown mustard seeds, whole (omit for Pitta)

¼ teaspoon freshly ground black pepper

½ cup of raw, unsalted cashew pieces

2 tablespoons finely minced fresh ginger

1 carrot, thinly sliced

1 zucchini, chopped

1 yellow squash, chopped

4 crimini mushrooms, sliced

½ red bell pepper, chopped

2 tablespoons shredded coconut (use 1 tablespoon for kapha), plus for garnish

2 scallions (white and green parts), chopped, plus for garnish

¼ cup chopped cilantro leaves, plus for garnish

Juice of 1 lime

¼ teaspoon salt

¼ cup Spicy Stir-Fry Sauce (page 185)

**To make the quinoa**

1. In a large saucepan, boil the water. Add the quinoa, coconut oil, turmeric, and salt. Reduce the heat to medium-low and cook, mostly covered, for 15 minutes, stirring every 5 minutes.

2. Turn off the heat, but keep the pan on the hot burner. Cover completely until needed.

**To make the stir-fry**

1. In a large, deep sauté pan or skillet, heat the coconut oil over medium heat. Add the cumin seeds, brown mustard seeds, and black pepper. Sauté for 2 minutes, stirring frequently.

2. Add the cashews and ginger, and sauté for 1 minute more, stirring frequently.

3. Add the carrot, zucchini, yellow squash, mushrooms, and bell pepper. Stir well. Reduce the heat slightly to medium-low and sauté, uncovered, for 5 minutes, stirring every 2 minutes.

4. Add the coconut and sauté for 1 minute more, stirring constantly.

5. Cover the pan and remove it from the heat.

6. Add the cooked quinoa to the sautéed veggies and stir well. If needed, you can transfer these ingredients into a large mixing bowl.

7. Stir in the scallions, cilantro, lime juice, salt, and stir-fry sauce, and blend well.

8. Garnish each bowl with additional scallions, coconut, and cilantro.

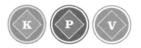

# Sweet Potato and Kale Quinoa Scramble

**GOOD FOR:** Digestion, Energy, Constipation, Heart Health, Skin Health, Eye Health, Pregnancy, Postpartum

**SERVES 3 TO 4 / PREP TIME: 5 MINUTES / COOK TIME: 25 MINUTES**

This quick and delicious dinner is a meal your whole family can enjoy. Together, these wholesome ingredients offer a full range of protein, fiber, vitamins, minerals, and antioxidants, providing you with a healthy and nourishing meal to end your busy day.

**For the quinoa**

2 cups water

1 cup quinoa

1 tablespoon sunflower oil (use sesame for Vata)

⅛ teaspoon Tridoshic Masala (page 179)

⅛ teaspoon salt

1 tablespoon Spicy Stir-Fry Sauce (page 185)

**For the scramble**

3 tablespoons sunflower oil, divided (use sesame for Vata)

¼ cup onion minced

½ teaspoon cumin seeds, whole

½ teaspoon brown mustard seeds, whole (omit for Pitta)

¼ teaspoon freshly ground black pepper

1 teaspoon Tridoshic Masala (page 179)

Pinch cayenne pepper (optional; omit for Pitta)

¼ cup water

3 kale leaves, stemmed and chopped (use 1 cup for Vata)

1 small sweet potato, chopped (about 2 cups) (use 1 cup for Kapha)

3 eggs (optional; use 1 egg and 3 egg whites for Pitta and Kapha)

3 tablespoons Spicy Stir-Fry Sauce (page 185)

⅛ teaspoon salt

Chopped scallions (green parts), for garnish

**To make the quinoa**

1. In a medium saucepan, bring the water to a boil.

2. Add the quinoa, sunflower oil, Tridoshic Masala, and salt. Reduce the heat to medium-low and cook, mostly covered, for 15 minutes, stirring every 5 minutes.

3. Take the pan off the hot burner. Add 1 tablespoon of stir-fry sauce and stir well. Cover the pan and set aside.

**To make the scramble**

1. In a large, deep sauté pan or skillet, heat 2 tablespoons of sunflower oil over medium heat. Add the onion, cumin seeds, brown mustard seeds, and black pepper. Sauté for 2 minutes, stirring frequently.

2. Add the Tridoshic Masala and cayenne pepper (if using). Sauté for 30 seconds, stirring constantly.

3. Add the water, kale, and sweet potato. Cover the pan and sauté for 5 to 7 minutes over medium-low heat, stirring frequently. You will know the veggies are done when the kale is moist and tender and the sweet potato is soft all the way through.

4. When the vegetables are cooked, cover the pan and set aside.

5. In a small bowl, whisk the eggs (if using) well.

6. In a sauté pan, heat the remaining 1 tablespoon of sunflower oil over medium heat. Add the eggs and cook, whisking frequently for about 2 minutes, or until the eggs are fully cooked but still moist.

7. Add the cooked eggs and quinoa to the kale and sweet potato mixture in the sauté pan. Combine well.

8. Add the stir-fry sauce and salt. Stir well.

9. Serve topped with a handful of scallions. Add any extra stir-fry sauce, salt, or pepper if desired.

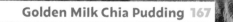
**Golden Milk Chia Pudding 167**

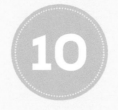

# DESSERTS

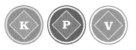

# Saffron Spiced Laddu

**GOOD FOR:** Energy, Mood-Enhancement, Complexion, Women's Reproductive Health, Libido, Pregnancy, Postpartum, Lactation

**MAKES 20 COOKIES / PREP TIME: 15 MINUTES / COOK TIME: 10 MINUTES / REST TIME: 30 MINUTES TO 2 HOURS**

Traditional Indian ball-shaped cookies, laddus are easy to make on the stovetop. This laddu recipe combines the healing powers of saffron along with chickpea flour as a base. Saffron is known for its ability to boost the mood, and promote happiness, peace, love, and compassion.

1 tablespoon cashews, finely ground (omit for Kapha)

1 tablespoon shredded coconut, finely ground (omit for Kapha)

¾ cup ghee

2 cups chickpea flour

½ teaspoon ground cinnamon

¼ teaspoon cardamom powder

⅛ teaspoon ground ginger (use ½ teaspoon for Kapha)

⅛ teaspoon turmeric powder

1 teaspoon saffron (about ½ gram), freshly ground

½ cup maple syrup (use honey for Kapha)

½ cup shredded coconut, for topping

**1.** Grind the cashews and the coconut in a spice grinder or blender and set aside until needed.

**2.** In a deep sauté pan or skillet, heat the ghee over medium heat until melted.

**3.** Reduce the heat to medium-low and stir in the chickpea flour.

**4.** Cook for 7 minutes, stirring continuously.

**5.** Add the cashews and coconut. Blend well. Continue to cook for 3 to 5 minutes more, or until the chickpea flour has become light brown and gives off a delicious aroma.

**6.** Transfer the batter into a large mixing bowl. Let it cool in the refrigerator for 5 minutes.

**7.** Add the cinnamon, cardamom, ginger, turmeric, saffron, and maple syrup. Blend well.

**8.** Take a small amount of the dough and roll it into a ball. If the mixture is sticky, wet your hands for a smoother roll; if the mixture is crumbly, add more melted ghee or maple syrup in very small increments.

**9.** Place the rolled ball onto a plate and continue to roll the batter until it is used up.

**10.** Place the shredded coconut in a small bowl. Roll each ball in the coconut, coating evenly.

**11.** Before eating, let the laddus cool at room temperature for 1 to 2 hours, or refrigerate them for 30 minutes. The finished cookie should not be sticky, gooey, or fall apart, but firm with a creamy softness (similar to a truffle).

**12.** Store in an airtight container at room temperature for 7 days or in the refrigerator for 2 to 3 weeks.

**INGREDIENT TIP:**
*You can find chickpea flour online; otherwise, replace it with equal amounts of whole wheat flour, coconut flour, or almond flour.*

# Sweet Sesame Laddu

**GOOD FOR:** Energy, Libido, Bone Health, Brain Health, Heart Health, Anemia, Women's Health, Pregnancy, Lactation, Postpartum, Menopause

**MAKES 25 TO 30 BALLS / PREP TIME: 30 MINUTES / CHILL TIME: 1 TO 2 HOURS**

These tasty treats are supportive for women's health, and with their powerful Ojas-enhancing properties, they will increase energy, strength, libido, and overall vitality.

¼ cup Tridoshic Almond Milk (page 57)

3 medjool dates, pitted and chopped

⅓ cup honey

2 teaspoons vanilla extract

1 teaspoon ground cinnamon

½ teaspoon ground ginger

¼ teaspoon cardamom powder

⅛ teaspoon turmeric powder

⅛ teaspoon salt

1 cup raw tahini

1 cup almonds

½ cup walnuts

¼ cup hemp seeds

¼ cup shredded coconut

2 tablespoons raw sesame seeds, plus ½ cup for coating

1. Put the almond milk, dates, honey, vanilla, cinnamon, ginger, cardamom, turmeric, and salt in a wide mouth jar. Using a hand blender, blend these ingredients into a thick, smooth paste. Alternatively, you can use a food processor or blender.

2. Transfer the liquid into a large mixing bowl and add the tahini. Blend well.

3. Put the almonds, walnuts, and hemp seeds into a blender. Blend on high for 1 to 2 minutes or until a coarse powder is formed.

4. Add the ground nuts and seeds, coconut, and raw sesame seeds to the date mixture. Using wet, clean hands, mix everything together.

5. Roll a small amount of batter in the palms of your hands. Place the completed ball onto a plate and continue to roll the batter until it is used up. The batter will be sticky; wet your hands between rolls to prevent sticking.

6. Put ½ cup of sesame seeds in a small bowl.

7. Roll each ball in the sesame seeds until fully coated.

8. Place the balls in the freezer for 1 to 2 hours before serving.

9. Store in an airtight container in the freezer for up to 3 months.

**TASTY TIP:**

*Create energizing chocolate sesame laddus by adding 2 tablespoons of cacao powder or cocoa powder to the blended ingredients (step 3).*

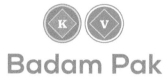

# Badam Pak

**GOOD FOR:** Energy, Women's Reproductive Health, Libido, Pregnancy, Postpartum, Lactation

**MAKES 16 BARS / PREP TIME: 15 MINUTES / COOK TIME: 10 MINUTES / CHILL TIME: 30 MINUTES TO 2 HOURS**

Badam Pak is a sweet bar that nourishes the mind and body. This irresistible recipe combines the health benefits of almonds with chickpea flour, ghee, aromatic spices, and coconut to make a life-promoting, nutrient-packed snack and oh-so-healthy dessert.

---

1½ cups almonds

¾ cup ghee

1 teaspoon vanilla extract

1 cup chickpea flour

¼ cup shredded coconut

½ cup honey

1 teaspoon ground cinnamon, plus for topping

½ teaspoon ground ginger

⅛ teaspoon cardamom powder

½ teaspoon saffron, freshly ground

Shredded coconut, for topping

---

**1.** Put the almonds in a blender or food processor, and blend on high for 1 to 2 minutes, or until a coarse powder is formed. It is all right to have some chunks, because this adds a pleasant crunchiness to the bars.

**2.** In a large, deep sauté pan or skillet, heat the ghee over medium heat until melted.

**3.** Reduce the heat to medium-low and stir in the vanilla.

**4.** Add the ground almonds and chickpea flour. Blend the dry ingredients with the ghee until a moist batter has been formed.

**5.** Stirring continuously, cook for 7 minutes.

**6.** Add the coconut. Stir until everything is evenly blended. Continue to cook for 1 to 2 minutes more, stirring constantly.

**7.** Place the batter into a large mixing bowl. Refrigerate for 5 minutes to cool.

**8.** Add the honey, cinnamon, ginger, cardamom, and saffron. Blend evenly.

**9.** Place a piece of parchment paper in an 8-by-8-inch baking dish.

**10.** Add the batter and flatten out evenly.

**11.** Sprinkle shredded coconut over the top, and dust with ground cinnamon.

**12.** Cover the baking dish and place it in the refrigerator for 1 to 2 hours or the freezer for 30 minutes. The finished bars should not be sticky, gooey, or fall apart, but firm with a slight softness.

**13.** Cut the bars into squares and place them in an airtight container. They will keep fresh in the refrigerator for up to 3 weeks.

**+ HEALTH TIP:**

*To make these bars even more rejuvenating, add 2 tablespoons of ashwagandha powder for men or 2 tablespoons of shatavari powder for women.*

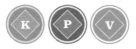

# Quick and Easy Quinoa Kheer

**GOOD FOR:** Energy, Immunity, Libido, Constipation, Anxiety, Pregnancy, Postpartum, Lactation

**SERVES 4 TO 6 / PREP TIME: 5 MINUTES (PLUS 30 MINUTES TO SOAK, OPTIONAL) / COOK TIME: 25 MINUTES**

Kheer is a simple, creamy Indian rice pudding. This variation uses quinoa rather than the traditional basmati rice, replaces some of the milk with water, and contains extra spices such as cinnamon, ginger, and turmeric. It is generally best to eat kheer during the fall and winter seasons because it is grounding, nourishing, slightly sweet, and very soothing on a cold day.

1 cup quinoa

8 to 10 saffron threads

¾ cup water

2 cups whole milk or Tridoshic Almond Milk (page 57, use almond milk for Kapha)

2 teaspoons ghee, divided (omit for Kapha)

2 cinnamon sticks

⅛ teaspoon pink Himalayan salt

Cashew pieces, for garnish (optional; omit for Kapha)

Shredded coconut, for garnish (omit for Kapha)

30 raisins

½ teaspoon ground cinnamon

¼ teaspoon ground ginger (use ½ teaspoon for Kapha), plus for garnish

⅛ teaspoon cardamom powder

⅛ teaspoon turmeric powder

1 teaspoon vanilla extract

Honey, for serving (use maple syrup for Pitta)

1. Soak the quinoa for a minimum of 30 minutes before cooking. Drain and discard the water before use.

2. Soak the saffron for 10 minutes in ¾ cup of water. Do not drain the water, because it will be added to the recipe.

3. In a large saucepan, heat the water and milk until just under a boil.

4. Reduce the heat to low and add the quinoa, 1 teaspoon of ghee, the cinnamon sticks, salt, and soaked saffron and soaking water. Stir well.

5. Cook, mostly covered, on medium-low for 20 minutes. Stir every 4 to 5 minutes.

6. While the quinoa is cooking, warm a small sauté pan over medium heat and dry roast the cashew pieces (if using) and coconut. Stirring constantly, sauté for 1 to 3 minutes, or until the coconut turns a light tan color. Set aside.

7. Once the quinoa is cooked, turn the heat off, but leave the saucepan on the warm burner. The kheer should be slightly soupy with a small amount of extra liquid, which will thicken upon sitting.

8. Add the raisins, the remaining 1 teaspoon of ghee, the cinnamon, ginger, cardamom, turmeric, and vanilla. Cover the pan and let sit for 5 minutes.

9. Serve in small bowls as a light, sweet, and creamy dessert or a wholesome snack. After the pudding has cooled slightly, add 1 to 2 teaspoons of honey per serving. Top with the coconut and cashews (if using), and sprinkle with cinnamon.

10. Eat, nourish, and enjoy in good company.

# Winter-Spiced Rice Pudding

**GOOD FOR:** Energy, Libido, Constipation, Bone Health, Colon Health, Pregnancy, Postpartum, Lactation

**SERVES 4 / PREP TIME: 5 MINUTES / COOK TIME: 25 MINUTES**

Looking for a dessert to keep you warm on those cold winter days? This comforting dish will make you want to cuddle up with a blanket and watch the snow fall.

3 cups water, divided

2 cups milk

1 cup basmati rice

2 teaspoons ghee, divided

2 cinnamon sticks

½ teaspoon salt

4 saffron threads

1 teaspoon ground cinnamon, plus for garnish

¼ teaspoon ground ginger

⅛ teaspoon cardamom powder

¼ cup shredded coconut, plus for garnish

2 heaping tablespoons raisins

1 teaspoon vanilla extract

2 to 4 tablespoons maple syrup

1. In a large saucepan, heat 2 cups of water and the milk until just under a boil.

2. Reduce the heat to low and add the rice, 1 teaspoon of ghee, the cinnamon sticks, salt, and saffron. Stir well.

3. Cook, mostly covered, for 25 minutes. Stir every 4 to 5 minutes.

4. Turn the heat off but leave the pan on the warm burner.

5. Add the remaining 1 cup of water, the remaining 1 teaspoon of ghee, the cinnamon, ginger, cardamom, coconut, raisins, and vanilla. Stir well.

6. Stir in 2 tablespoons of maple syrup. Give a quick taste, and if more syrup is needed, add 1 to 2 tablespoons more depending on your preference.

7. Cover the pan and let the pudding sit for 5 minutes to allow it to soften and the flavors to harmonize.

8. Serve warm in small bowls and top with a handful of coconut and a sprinkle of cinnamon.

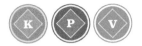

# Golden Milk Chia Pudding

**GOOD FOR:** Energy, Digestion, Constipation, Weight Loss, Inflammation, Colon Health, Bone Health, Heart Health, Skin Health, Hair Health, Pregnancy, Postpartum, Lactation

**SERVES 2 TO 3 / PREP TIME: 10 MINUTES / CHILL TIME: 1 TO 3 HOURS**

This Golden Milk Chia Pudding combines the powers of chia seeds with the healing properties of turmeric to create a delicious treat. It is a great dessert option when you're trying to lose weight because it will sustain your sweet tooth without creating heaviness.

1½ cups Tridoshic Almond Milk (page 57)

3 dates, pitted and chopped (use 2 dates for Kapha)

1 tablespoon honey (use maple syrup for Pitta)

½ teaspoon ground cinnamon

¼ teaspoon ground ginger

¼ teaspoon turmeric powder

⅛ teaspoon cardamom powder

1 teaspoon vanilla extract

4 tablespoons chia seeds

2 to 6 teaspoons shredded coconut, divided

1. Put the almond milk, dates, honey, cinnamon, ginger, turmeric, cardamom, and vanilla in a blender. Blend on high for 1 to 2 minutes, or until a thick and creamy consistency has been reached.

2. Put the almond milk blend in a pint-size glass jar with a lid. Add the chia seeds.

3. Stir well, making sure all the chia seeds become immersed in the liquid.

4. Let sit for 15 minutes, stirring every 5 minutes.

5. Refrigerate the chia blend. The chia pudding can be eaten as soon as 1 hour after making this recipe; however, it is best to wait at least 2 to 3 hours.

6. Stir the pudding before serving in small bowls.

7. Stir 1 to 2 teaspoons of shredded coconut into each serving directly before eating. This will allow the coconut to stay crisp and add a pleasant texture.

# Avocado, Coconut, and Cacao Pudding

**SERVES 2 TO 4 / PREP TIME: 10 MINUTES / CHILL TIME: 1 HOUR (OPTIONAL)**

If you think healthy eating can't be delicious, quick, and easy, you haven't tried this recipe! This superfood pudding boasts incredibly rejuvenating, mind-boosting, Ojas-enhancing properties for Pitta and Vata types to indulge in throughout the late spring and summer seasons.

2 medium, ripe avocados

2 tablespoons cacao powder (use 1 tablespoon for Vata)

3 tablespoons maple syrup

1 teaspoon vanilla extract

¾ cup coconut water, divided

Shredded coconut, for garnish

1. Scoop the meat out of the avocados. Put the avocado in a bowl if you are using a hand blender, or if you are using a regular blender, put the avocado directly into the blender.

2. Add the cacao powder, maple syrup, vanilla, and ½ cup of the coconut water.

3. Blend on high until the mixture is smooth and there are no chunks. If the pudding seems too thick, add the remaining ¼ cup of coconut water and blend again.

4. Transfer the pudding to a covered bowl and refrigerate. Let the mixture chill for at least 1 hour before serving (optional, but recommended).

5. Serve sprinkled with the coconut.

6. Indulge and energize! Enjoy this treat as a decadent snack or healthy dessert.

# Heavenly Hummus Chocolate Pudding

**GOOD FOR:** Energy, Appetite Control, Constipation, Anemia, Bone Health, Colon Health, Cancer Prevention, Postpartum

**SERVES 2 / PREP TIME: 10 MINUTES (PLUS 15 TO 25 MINUTES TO SOAK)**

If you are craving a rich, chocolatey, mousse-like dessert, this pudding delivers! This surprisingly decadent recipe becomes a protein-packed, nutritious treat that will power you through your day. Although sweets can be provoking for Kapha, the chickpeas and honey balance out this dosha.

3 medjool dates, pitted
(use 1 date for Kapha)

¾ cup coconut water, divided

1 to 2 tablespoons honey
(use maple syrup for Pitta)

1 teaspoon vanilla extract

½ teaspoon ground cinnamon

¼ teaspoon cardamom powder

¼ teaspoon ground ginger

⅛ teaspoon salt

2 tablespoons tahini

3 tablespoons cacao powder

1 can chickpeas (1½ cups cooked)

1. Soak the pitted dates in ½ cup coconut water for 15 to 25 minutes.

2. Put the soaked dates, ½ cup of the soaked coconut water, honey, vanilla, cinnamon, cardamom, ginger, salt, tahini, and cacao into a blender.

3. Blend on high for 1 to 2 minutes, or until a thick, smooth, creamy consistency has been reached.

4. Add the chickpeas and blend on high for 2 to 3 minutes more. Make sure there are no chunks remaining. If the pudding seems too thick, stir in the remaining ¼ cup of soaked coconut water and blend again.

5. This chocolate hummus will last in an airtight container in the refrigerator for up to 5 days.

# Irresistible Carrot Cake Muffins

**GOOD FOR:** Energy, Skin Health, Eye Health, Colon Health, Pregnancy, Postpartum, Lactation

**MAKES 12 MUFFINS / PREP TIME: 15 MINUTES / COOK TIME: 15 MINUTES**

These extra-moist Irresistible Carrot Cake Muffins may become a staple to have around your home during the fall and winter seasons. They combine the deliciousness of muffins with the health-promoting powers of carrots and whole wheat. This recipe becomes even more healing with the addition of warming spices, ghee, and a small amount of maple syrup (no sugar needed!).

**For the muffins**

1⅔ cups of 100 percent whole wheat flour

1 teaspoon baking soda

1 teaspoon baking powder

2 teaspoons ground cinnamon

½ teaspoon ground ginger

¼ teaspoon cardamom powder

¼ teaspoon turmeric powder

¼ teaspoon salt

2 eggs

½ cup maple syrup

¼ cup melted ghee or coconut oil

½ cup plain yogurt

1 teaspoon vanilla extract

2 cups grated carrots
(about 4 carrots)

**For the topping**

1 tablespoon melted ghee

1 tablespoon honey

¼ teaspoon ground cinnamon

**To make the muffins**

1. Preheat the oven to 375°F.

2. In a large mixing bowl, combine the flour, baking soda, baking powder, cinnamon, ginger, cardamom, turmeric, and salt.

3. In a medium mixing bowl, combine the eggs, maple syrup, ghee, yogurt, and vanilla. Whisk thoroughly until completely blended.

4. Add the wet ingredients to the dry ingredients. Stir until everything is evenly moist and blended.

5. Fold in the grated carrots, making sure to combine them evenly without overmixing.

6. Oil a nonstick 12-count muffin pan (or use muffin liners).

7. Fill each muffin pan with ¼ cup of batter.

8. Bake for 14 to 16 minutes, until the tops are golden brown and a toothpick comes out clean. You will know they are done if you press lightly in the center and the muffin springs back.

9. Let cool before adding the topping and serving.

**To make the topping**

1. Warm the ghee slightly, just enough to become liquid but not hot.

2. In a small bowl, combine the ghee, honey, and cinnamon.

3. Once the muffins are cool, use a small spoon to drizzle a tiny amount of the topping onto the center of each muffin, allowing the liquid to slightly drip down, covering the top and sides of the muffins.

4. These muffins taste great alongside the Masala Chai (page 55) on a cold winter or fall day.

# Chocolate Chip Cookies

**GOOD FOR:** Energy, Rejuvenation, Pregnancy, Postpartum

**MAKES 24 COOKIES / PREP TIME: 15 MINUTES / COOK TIME: 15 MINUTES**

These cookies are made with whole wheat flour, ghee, and warming spices to enhance digestion. They are sweetened with maple syrup and dark chocolate chips. The result is a sweet, nourishing treat your whole family will love!

2 cups of 100 percent whole wheat flour

½ teaspoon baking soda

¼ teaspoon ground cinnamon

¼ teaspoon ground ginger

⅛ teaspoon cardamom powder

⅛ teaspoon turmeric powder

½ teaspoon salt

2 eggs

½ cup maple syrup

1 tablespoon molasses

½ cup melted ghee

1 teaspoon vanilla extract

1 cup dark chocolate chips (optional; omit for Vata imbalance)

1. Preheat the oven to 325°F.

2. In a large mixing bowl, combine the flour, baking soda, cinnamon, ginger, cardamom, turmeric, and salt.

3. In a medium mixing bowl, combine the eggs, maple syrup, molasses, ghee, and vanilla. Whisk thoroughly.

4. Add the wet ingredients to the dry ingredients. Using an electric mixer, mix on medium until well blended.

5. Fold in the chocolate chips (if using) with a large spoon.

6. Place parchment paper onto two cookie sheets. Roll the dough into small balls. Place 12 balls onto each cookie sheet, spacing them evenly.

7. Bake for 10 minutes, until golden brown.

8. Cool the cookies on a wire rack.

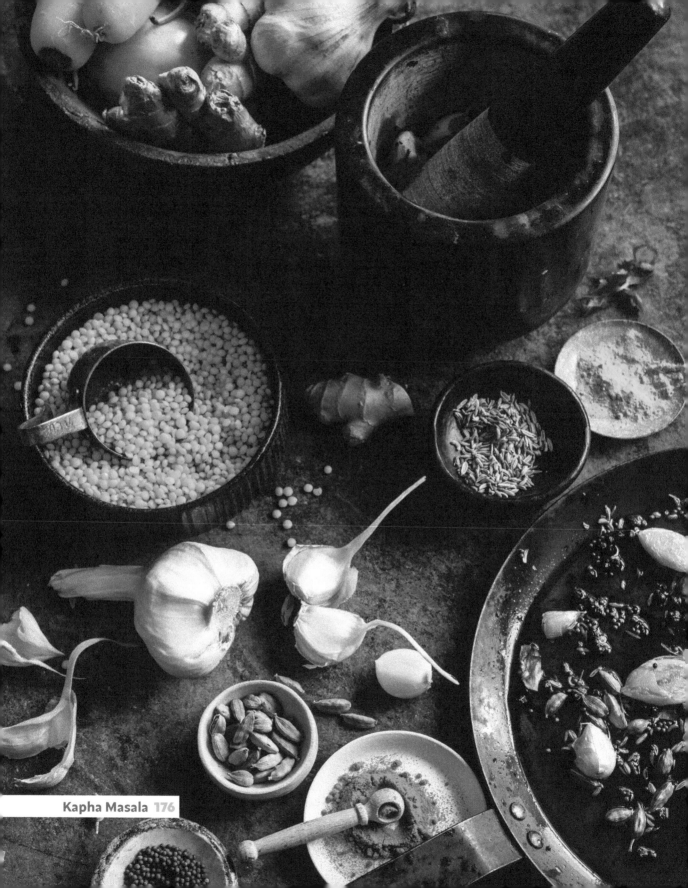

Kapha Masala **176**

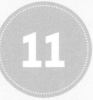

# CONDIMENTS, SAUCES, AND SPICE BLENDS

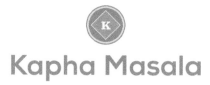

# Kapha Masala

**GOOD FOR:** Digestion, Absorption, Detox, Metabolism, Weight Loss, Circulation

### MAKES 1 CUP / PREP TIME: 10 MINUTES

This spice blend will help treat all Kapha digestive issues such as slow digestion, slow metabolism, weight gain, and lethargy after meals. You can add it to any savory food or recipe to enhance flavor and digestibility. This heating, stimulating blend helps make heavy foods less heavy and boosts digestive fire all around. To get the full effects of the spice blend, dry roast it for 30 to 60 seconds before adding it to your food.

5 tablespoons turmeric powder

5 tablespoons ground ginger

3 tablespoons cumin seeds, whole

2 tablespoons brown mustard seeds, whole

2 tablespoons ground cinnamon

1 tablespoon black peppercorns, whole

1 tablespoon cardamom powder

10 cloves

1. Put the turmeric, ginger, cumin seeds, brown mustard seeds, cinnamon, peppercorns, cardamom, and cloves into a blender, and blend on high for 1 to 3 minutes to form a powder.

2. Transfer the spice mixture to a bowl and stir it to blend evenly.

3. Label and store the masala in an airtight jar.

### INGREDIENT TIP:

*The turmeric powder or Tridoshic Masala (page 179) in any recipe can be replaced with equal amounts of the Kapha Masala.*

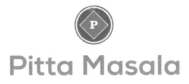

# Pitta Masala

**GOOD FOR:** Digestion, Absorption, Hyperacidity, Acid Reflux, Heartburn, Detox, Inflammation, Liver Health

**MAKES 1 CUP / PREP TIME: 10 MINUTES**

This spice blend will help treat all Pitta digestive issues such as acid reflux, heartburn, inflammation in the GI tract, and loose stools. This blend also works to cool down foods that may typically be too heating for Pitta types. To get the full effects of this blend, sauté it in ghee or coconut oil for about 30 to 60 seconds before adding it to your food.

4 tablespoons turmeric powder

4 tablespoons ground ginger

3 tablespoons fennel seeds, whole

3 tablespoons coriander seeds, whole

2 tablespoons cumin seeds, whole

1 tablespoon cardamom powder

**1.** Put the turmeric, ginger, fennel seeds, coriander seeds, cumin seeds, and cardamom into a blender, and blend on high for 1 to 3 minutes to form a powder.

**2.** Transfer the spice mixture to a bowl and stir it to blend evenly.

**3.** Label and store the masala in an airtight jar.

**INGREDIENT TIP:**

*The turmeric powder or Tridoshic Masala (page 179) listed in these recipes can be replaced with equal amounts of the Pitta Masala.*

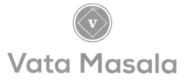

# Vata Masala

**GOOD FOR:** Digestion, Absorption, Gas, Bloating, Constipation, Detox, Inflammation

**MAKES 1 CUP / PREP TIME: 10 MINUTES**

This spice blend helps pacify common Vata digestive issues such as gas, bloating, and constipation. It works in any savory recipe to enhance flavor and health properties. To experience the full effects of the spice blend, first sauté it in ghee or sesame oil for 30 to 60 seconds before adding it to your food.

4 tablespoons turmeric powder

4 tablespoons ground ginger

3 tablespoons cumin seeds, whole

2 tablespoons ground cinnamon

2 tablespoons fennel seeds, whole

1 tablespoon fenugreek seeds, whole

1 tablespoon black peppercorns, whole

1 teaspoon mineral salt or pink Himalayan salt

¼ teaspoon hing (if available)

1. Put the turmeric, ginger, cumin seeds, cinnamon, fennel seeds, fenugreek seeds, peppercorns, salt, and hing (if using) into a blender, and blend on high for 1 to 3 minutes to form a powder.

2. Transfer the spice mixture to a bowl and stir it to blend evenly.

3. Label and store the masala in an airtight jar.

### INGREDIENT TIP:

*The turmeric powder or Tridoshic Masala (page 179) listed in these recipes can be replaced with equal amounts of the Vata Masala.*

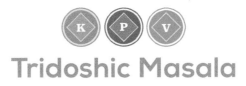

# Tridoshic Masala

**MAKES 1½ CUPS / PREP TIME: 10 MINUTES**

This tridoshic blend will enhance digestive fire without creating excessive heat in the body. It can be added to any savory food or recipe to improve digestion, promote absorption of nutrients, enhance metabolism, increase circulation, burn toxins, and prevent symptoms of indigestion such as gas and bloating. To get the full effects of the spice mixture, sauté it in ghee or oil for 30 to 60 seconds before adding it to your food.

5 tablespoons turmeric powder

5 tablespoons ground ginger

4 tablespoons cumin seeds, whole

4 tablespoons fennel seeds, whole

4 tablespoons coriander seeds, whole

1 tablespoon brown mustard seeds, whole (omit for Pitta)

1 tablespoon fenugreek seeds, whole

1 tablespoon black peppercorns, whole

1 tablespoon cardamom powder

1. Put the turmeric, ginger, cumin seeds, fennel seeds, coriander seeds, brown mustard seeds, fenugreek seeds, peppercorns, and cardamom into a blender, and blend on high for 1 to 3 minutes to form a powder.

2. Transfer the spice mixture to a bowl and stir it to blend evenly.

3. Label and store the masala in an airtight jar.

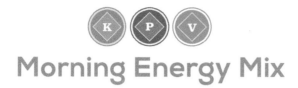

# Morning Energy Mix

**GOOD FOR:** Energy, Heart Health, Skin Health, Hair Health, Brain Health, Cancer Prevention, Postpartum

**MAKES 1 CUP / PREP TIME: 10 MINUTES**

Here is a unique blend of seeds, coconut, and cacao that will enhance any breakfast or smoothie recipe and leave you energized and ready to take on the day! This delicious blend adds a bit of creaminess to your oatmeal and porridges, and thanks to a strong dose of cacao powder, it is sure to add a whole lot of flavor, too.

¼ cup flaxseed, whole
(use ½ cup for Kapha)

¼ cup hemp seeds

¼ cup cacao powder
(use 1 to 2 tablespoons for Vata)

½ cup shredded coconut
(use ¼ cup for Kapha)

1. Put the flaxseed into a blender and blend on high to form a powder.

2. Add the hemp seeds, cacao, and coconut to the blender.

3. Blend on high for 1 to 2 minutes, or until all the ingredients have been ground into a thick, paste-like consistency. Stir periodically while blending if needed.

4. Transfer the mixture to a bowl and stir it to blend evenly.

5. Store in an airtight jar. This keeps in the refrigerator for up to 1 month, but is best used within 1 week.

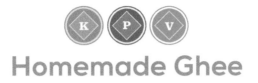

# Homemade Ghee

**GOOD FOR:** Digestion, Detox, Energy, Inflammation, Constipation, Nervous System Health, Pregnancy, Postpartum, Lactation

**MAKES 2 CUPS / COOK TIME: 20 TO 30 MINUTES**

Ghee is an Ayurvedic staple. It is a healthy alternative for oil or butter and is added to many dishes to enhance flavor. Although you can buy ghee in many natural grocery stores, making it at home will provide you with a fresher ghee and more powerful health benefits.

1 pound (4 sticks) unsalted, organic butter

1. In a medium saucepan, heat the butter over medium heat, stirring occasionally.

2. Once the butter has melted, reduce the heat to low.

3. Let the melted butter sit, uncovered, on low heat for 20 minutes. A frothy white foam will begin to form on top; this represents the milk solids separating from the oil, and can be removed with a clean, dry spoon periodically (optional).

4. The cooking process is complete when the cloudiness of the original butter disappears and you are able to see through the liquid. It should resemble a translucent oil. The white foam will settle at the bottom of the pan.

5. Once the ghee is completely transparent and the curds at the bottom begin to brown just slightly, remove the pan from the heat.

6. Remove the remaining milk solids by straining the finished ghee into a clean and dry glass container. This can be done by using a cheesecloth or a thick paper towel placed over a fine-mesh strainer.

7. The ghee will become solid once it cools to room temperature. If the weather is warm, it may stay liquid or semiliquid.

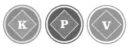

# Digestion-Enhancing Ginger Syrup

**GOOD FOR:** Digestion, Detox, Constipation, Gas, Bloating, Weight Loss, Inflammation, Immunity, Congestion, Nausea, Morning Sickness, Pregnancy, Postpartum, Menstrual Cramps

**MAKES 1 CUP / PREP TIME: 15 MINUTES**

This syrup is quick to prepare and contains only four ingredients. It enhances digestion, speeds metabolism, and helps flush out toxins. The ingredients will also aid in weight loss, reduce inflammation, alleviate nausea and morning sickness, increase immunity, clear congestion, and relieve menstrual cramping.

½ cup honey

¼ cup fresh lime juice (about 2 limes)

½ cup peeled and finely minced fresh ginger

⅛ teaspoon pink Himalayan or mineral salt

1. Put the honey, lime juice, ginger, and salt into a blender.

2. Blend on medium for 1 to 2 minutes. The ingredients should get evenly mixed and the consistency will be like a thick syrup. The ginger will not blend completely but should become a fine, pulp-like texture.

3. Pour the syrup into a glass jar with a lid.

4. Take 1 to 2 teaspoons of this digestive aid up to 15 minutes before each meal.

5. Store in an airtight jar in the refrigerator for 3 to 6 months.

# Coconut-Cilantro Chutney

**GOOD FOR:** Digestion, Detox, Excessive Heat, Inflammation, Liver Health, Skin Health, Allergies

**MAKES 1 CUP / PREP TIME: 15 TO 20 MINUTES**

Enhance any dal or kitchari recipe with this irresistible, flavorful chutney. Its cooling properties help dampen the heat from spicy meals, making them more Pitta-friendly. The lime, cilantro, ginger, and pepper increase the digestibility of the food, promote mild detoxification, and reduce inflammation.

1 tablespoon ghee

¼ teaspoon brown mustard seeds, whole (omit for Pitta)

½ teaspoon cumin seeds, whole

½ cup water

¼ cup fresh lime juice (about 2 limes)

¼ teaspoon pink Himalayan or mineral salt

1 tablespoon chopped ginger (1-inch cube)

1 to 2 teaspoons serrano pepper, chopped (omit for Pitta)

2 tablespoons cashew pieces

¾ packed cup finely chopped cilantro

¾ cup shredded coconut (use ⅓ cup for Kapha)

1. In a small sauté pan, heat the ghee over medium heat. Add the brown mustard seeds and cumin seeds. Sauté for 2 minutes, stirring frequently.

2. Put the water, lime juice, sautéed spices, salt, ginger, pepper, cashews, cilantro, and coconut into a blender. Blend on high for 1 to 3 minutes. Stir periodically while blending if needed. The ingredients should become evenly mixed and the consistency will have a creamy, slightly pulp-like texture. A small amount of water or lime juice (1 to 2 tablespoons) can be added if needed.

3. Transfer the chutney to a glass jar with a lid.

4. Store in an airtight jar in the refrigerator for up to 5 days.

# Golden Tahini Sauce

**GOOD FOR:** Bone Health, Anemia, Immunity, Inflammation, Pregnancy, Postpartum, Lactation

**MAKES 1¾ CUPS / PREP TIME: 5 MINUTES / COOK TIME: 5 MINUTES**

This deliciously creamy sauce will increase the health benefits of any dish by adding a substantial amount of calcium, magnesium, zinc, and iron. Turmeric provides a beautiful golden color.

1 teaspoon cumin seeds, whole

½ teaspoon brown mustard seeds, whole

½ teaspoon black peppercorns, whole

1 teaspoon sesame oil

1 teaspoon Vata Masala (page 178) or turmeric

1 cup tahini

1 cup Tridoshic Almond Milk (page 57)

1 tablespoon fresh lemon juice

½ teaspoon mineral or pink Himalayan salt

**1.** Put the cumin seeds, brown mustard seeds, and black peppercorns into a blender, and blend on high for 1 to 3 minutes to form a powder.

**2.** In a small sauté pan, heat the sesame oil over medium heat. Add the ground spices. Sauté for 1½ minutes, stirring frequently.

**3.** Reduce the heat to low. Add the Vata Masala (or turmeric) and cook for 30 seconds, stirring constantly.

**4.** Add the tahini and almond milk. Stir well. Warm over low heat for 3 minutes, stirring each minute.

**5.** Take the pan off the heat and mix in the lemon juice and salt.

**6.** Enjoy this sauce as a creamy condiment to any kitchari, dal, rice, vegetable, or quinoa recipe. This sauce can be used as a nourishing veggie dip or creamy spread, or paired with hummus recipes as well.

**7.** Refrigerate in an airtight container for up to 5 days.

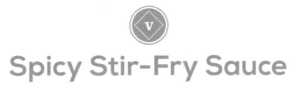

# Spicy Stir-Fry Sauce

**GOOD FOR:** Digestion

**MAKES 1 CUP / PREP TIME: 10 MINUTES**

This stir-fry sauce makes a great kitchen staple. It is a heating blend, but can be enjoyed in small amounts by all body types (with the appropriate modifications) and throughout all seasons. If you are on a low-sodium diet or experiencing more severe Pitta or Kapha issues, avoid this recipe.

¼ cup soy sauce

¼ cup fresh lime juice (about 2 limes)

2 tablespoons ume plum vinegar

2 tablespoons sesame oil (use sunflower oil for Kapha and Pitta)

½ teaspoon ground ginger

¼ teaspoon cayenne pepper (omit for Pitta)

1. Pour the soy sauce, lime juice, vinegar, and sesame oil into a pint-size jar.
2. Add the ground ginger and cayenne pepper.
3. Stir well using a spoon, or place a lid on the jar and shake thoroughly.
4. Store in an airtight jar for up to 3 months. Stir or shake this blend before each use to avoid separation.

# THE DIRTY DOZEN AND THE CLEAN FIFTEEN™

A nonprofit environmental watchdog organization called the Environmental Working Group (EWG) looks at data supplied by the US Department of Agriculture (USDA) and the Food and Drug Administration (FDA) about pesticide residues. Each year it compiles a list of the best and worst pesticide loads found in commercial crops. You can use these lists to decide which fruits and vegetables to buy organic to minimize your exposure to pesticides and which produce is considered safe enough to buy conventionally. This does not mean they are pesticide-free, though, so wash these fruits and vegetables thoroughly. The list is updated annually, and you can find it online at EWG.org/FoodNews.

## Dirty Dozen™

1. strawberries
2. spinach
3. kale
4. nectarines
5. apples
6. grapes
7. peaches
8. cherries
9. pears
10. tomatoes
11. celery
12. potatoes

†Additionally, nearly three-quarters of hot pepper samples contained pesticide residues.

## Clean Fifteen™

1. avocados
2. sweet corn*
3. pineapples
4. sweet peas (frozen)
5. onions
6. papayas*
7. eggplants
8. asparagus
9. kiwis
10. cabbages
11. cauliflower
12. cantaloupes
13. broccoli
14. mushrooms
15. honeydew melons

*A small amount of sweet corn, papaya, and summer squash sold in the United States is produced from genetically modified seeds. Buy organic varieties of these crops if you want to avoid genetically modified produce.

# MEASUREMENT CONVERSIONS

## Volume Equivalents (Liquid)

| US STANDARD | US STANDARD (OUNCES) | METRIC (APPROXIMATE) |
|---|---|---|
| 2 tablespoons | 1 fl. oz. | 30 mL |
| ¼ cup | 2 fl. oz. | 60 mL |
| ½ cup | 4 fl. oz. | 120 mL |
| 1 cup | 8 fl. oz. | 240 mL |
| 1½ cups | 12 fl. oz. | 355 mL |
| 2 cups or 1 pint | 16 fl. oz. | 475 mL |
| 4 cups or 1 quart | 32 fl. oz. | 1 L |
| 1 gallon | 128 fl. oz. | 4 L |

## Oven Temperatures

| FAHRENHEIT (F) | CELSIUS (C) (APPROXIMATE) |
|---|---|
| 250°F | 120°C |
| 300°F | 150°C |
| 325°F | 165°C |
| 350°F | 180°C |
| 375°F | 190°C |
| 400°F | 200°C |
| 425°F | 220°C |
| 450°F | 230°C |

## Volume Equivalents (Dry)

| US STANDARD | METRIC (APPROXIMATE) |
|---|---|
| ⅛ teaspoon | 0.5 mL |
| ¼ teaspoon | 1 mL |
| ½ teaspoon | 2 mL |
| ¾ teaspoon | 4 mL |
| 1 teaspoon | 5 mL |
| 1 tablespoon | 15 mL |
| ¼ cup | 59 mL |
| ⅓ cup | 79 mL |
| ½ cup | 118 mL |
| ⅔ cup | 156 mL |
| ¾ cup | 177 mL |
| 1 cup | 235 mL |
| 2 cups or 1 pint | 475 mL |
| 3 cups | 700 mL |
| 4 cups or 1 quart | 1 L |

## Weight Equivalents

| US STANDARD | METRIC (APPROXIMATE) |
|---|---|
| ½ ounce | 15 g |
| 1 ounce | 30 g |
| 2 ounces | 60 g |
| 4 ounces | 115 g |
| 8 ounces | 225 g |
| 12 ounces | 340 g |
| 16 ounces or 1 pound | 455 g |

# Ayurvedic Books

***Ayurveda: The Science of Self-healing : A Practical Guide* by Dr. Vasant Lad**, a basic introduction to Ayurveda for the beginner

***Balance Your Hormones, Balance Your Life* by Dr. Claudia Welch**, a book of healing from an Eastern perspective for beginner to experienced

***The Complete Book of Ayurvedic Home Remedies* by Dr. Vasant Lad**, for the beginner to the experienced practitioner, includes countless home remedies for ailments of all kinds

***Prakriti: Your Ayurvedic Constitution* by Dr. Robert Svoboda**, an introduction to the three doshas and your Ayurvedic body type for beginner to intermediate

***Textbook of Ayurveda, Volume 1* by Dr. Vasant Lad**, an in-depth introduction to Ayurveda for Ayurvedic students and practitioners

***The Yoga of Herbs: An Ayurvedic Guide to Herbal Medicine* by Dr. David Frawley and Dr. Vasant Lad**, a concise book on Ayurvedic herbs for beginner to intermediate

## Websites/Blogs

**Alandi Ashram:** http://ayurveda.alandiashram.org, an Ayurveda school and clinic in Boulder, Colorado, and online resource for Ayurvedic blog and recipes, from founders Alakananda Ma and Sadananda

**The Ayurvedic Institute:** https://www.ayurveda.com, an Ayurveda school and clinic in New Mexico and online resource for Ayurvedic video lectures, from founder Dr. Vasant Lad

**Ayurved Sadhana:** https://www.ayurvedsadhana.com, an Ayurveda school and clinic, from founders Dr. Bharat Vaidya and Anupama Vaidya

**Dr. Claudia Welch:** https://drclaudiawelch.com, an Ayurvedic doctor, teacher, and author, and an online resource with an Ayurveda blog, videos, and online Ayurvedic courses

**Dr. Robert Svoboda:** https://www.drsvoboda.com, an Ayurvedic doctor, teacher, and author, and online resource with an Ayurveda blog, videos, and online Ayurvedic courses

**Shadow Yoga:** https://shadowyoga.com, international Yoga training from founder Shandor Remete, cofounder Emma Balnaves

**Svastha Ayurveda:** https://svasthaayurveda.com, an online resource for handcrafted Ayurvedic herbal products, as well as an Ayurveda blog and recipes

# AILMENT INDEX

# INDEX

# ACKNOWLEDGMENTS

I would like to give great respect and thanks to all of my teachers, especially Alakananda Ma, Dr. Bharat Vaidya, Dr. Vasant Lad, Madeleine Huish, Shandor Remete, and Emma Balnaves. I am eternally grateful for their guidance and knowledge, which has helped shape me into the person I am today. I only hope I am able to keep up the integrity of their teachings and preserve the wisdom they hold. I thank my mom, Colleen Patterson, and pop, James Martin, my greatest teachers of them all! I thank my brother, Simon Martin, for his hard work, knowledge, and advice in my business and in life. I thank my family for helping me grow and evolve as an individual, for putting up with me throughout the highs and lows, and for allowing me to be myself (for better or for worse). And finally, I must give a huge thank-you to Nancy Paladino for being my right-hand lady throughout this crazy experience, as we cooked countless recipes, day in, day out, until we found "perfection."

## ABOUT THE AUTHOR

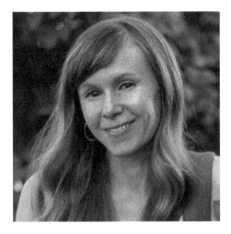

**Danielle Martin** is an Ayurvedic herbalist and practitioner. She is the founder of Svastha Ayurveda, an Ayurvedic herbal apothecary line. She graduated from the Ayurvedic Institute in 2011, and then went on to graduate from Alandi Ayurveda Gurukula in 2013 with her Ayurvedic Doctorate certification. She continues her studies at Ayurved Sadhana and is always excited to expand her knowledge. She is eternally grateful for her teachers of both Ayurveda and Yoga and does her best to keep the integrity of her studies strong.

Danielle currently lives in Boulder, Colorado, with her beautiful family of five. When she is not working, she enjoys a busy, but simple life cooking, reading, going for walks, practicing Yoga, and spending time with her family.

You can find her products and read more articles on her website at SvasthaAyurveda.com.

CPSIA information can be obtained
at www.ICGtesting.com
Printed in the USA
JSHW010142070321
12310JS00003B/10